Visit our website

to find out about other books from Churchill [Livingstone]
and our sister companies in Harcourt Health [Sciences]

Register free at
www.harcourt-international.com

and you will get

- **the latest information on new books, journals and electronic products in your chosen subject areas**

- **the choice of e-mail or post alerts or both, when there are any new books in your chosen areas**

- **news of special offers and promotions**

- **information about products from all Harcourt Health Sciences companies including Baillière Tindall, Churchill Livingstone, Mosby and W. B. Saunders**

You will also find an easily searchable catalogue, online ordering, information on our extensive list of journals...and much more!

Visit the Harcourt Health Sciences website today!

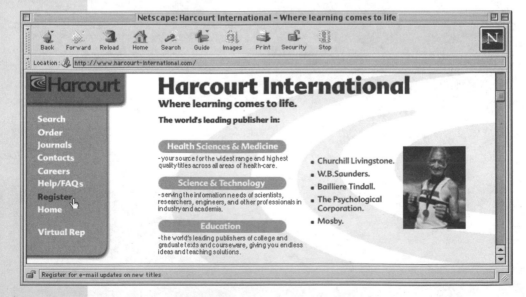

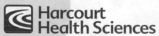

Caring for Sexuality in Health and Illness

For Churchill Livingstone:

Senior Commissioning Editor: Sarena Paisley
Project Development Manager: Karen Gilmour
Project Manager: Derek Robertson
Design Direction: George Ajayi

Caring for Sexuality in Health and Illness

Edited by

Diane Wells BA (Hons) RGN RNT Cassell Cert in Psychosocial Nursing
Lecturer, Faculty of Health and Social Care Sciences, Kingston University and
St George's Hospital Medical School, London

Authors:

Doreen Clifford RGN SCM MTD Cassell Cert in Psychosocial Nursing
Freelance Balint Leader for psychosexual seminars of health care professionals

Marjorie Rutter RGN FPCert FETC ENBAO8
Clinical Nurse Specialist, Family Planning and Well Woman Care,
King's College Hospital and Community Health, London;
Counsellor, Assisted Conception Unit, King's College Hospital, London

Jane Selby RGN FPCert FETC ENBAO8
Psychosexual Nurse Counsellor, Margaret Pyke Centre,
Camden and Islington Community Health Trust, London;
Freelance Balint Seminar Leader

Foreword by
Jan Savage
President of the Association of Psychosexual Nursing;
Author of *Nursing Intimacy*

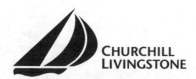

CHURCHILL LIVINGSTONE

EDINBURGH LONDON NEW YORK PHILADELPHIA ST LOUIS SYDNEY TORONTO 2000

CHURCHILL LIVINGSTONE
An imprint of Harcourt Publishers Limited

© Harcourt Publishers Limited 2000

_⁂_ is a registered trademark of Harcourt Publishers Limited

The rights of Diane Wells, Doreen Clifford, Marjorie Rutter and
Jane Selby to be identified as authors of this work have been asserted
by them in accordance with the Copyright, Designs and Patents Act
1988

First published 2000

ISBN 0443 06443 1

British Library Cataloguing in Publication Data
A catalogue record for this book is available from the British Library

Library of Congress Cataloging in Publication Data
A catalog record for this book is available from the Library of
Congress

The
publisher's
policy is to use
paper manufactured
from sustainable forests

Printed in the United Kingdom by Bell and Bain Ltd., Glasgow

Contents

Foreword

I am delighted to have been asked to write the foreword to this exciting and very timely book. Over the past ten to fifteen years there has been a steady increase in publications addressing issues associated with sexuality and health care. *Caring for Sexuality in Health and Illness* complements much of this previous work, but takes a very different stance. Part of the difference concerns the book's emphasis on the interdependence of practice and theory, and the opportunity it provides for reflection and active learning through the provision of a wide array of case examples. Underpinning this approach is a strong argument for Balint seminar training as a means of supporting health practitioners in recognizing and exploring their clients' psychosexual difficulties. Although not a new development, the work of Balint has contemporary relevance at a number of levels.

At the level of theory, through its emphasis on the emotions that lie at the heart of psychosexual problems and that re-emerge in practitioner/client interaction, Balint's work prefigures the burgeoning interest now evident among social scientists and others seeking to understand the links between emotions and health. In addition, the requirement of the practitioner to engage with emotions in an experiential way raises some interesting questions for those who wish to develop new research approaches that value and attempt to articulate lived experience, or new theoretical approaches that recognize non-rational forms of knowledge.

At the level of practice, Balint seminar training provides an arena in which practitioners can develop new understandings of their interactions with clients that can be used to inform future work. Such insights are often intuitive and tentative in nature. Sharing these insights with the client is not always easy, given that it means embracing a loss of certainty on the practitioner's behalf. Nevertheless, the advantages of such a stance include a challenge to traditional models of practice based on professional authority, and the promotion of a collaborative or negotiated approach to health care. Thus the forms of practice that develop from Balint training are arguably very much in keeping with the 'modernisation' of the National Health Service and with those policy initiatives that promote greater partnership between clients and health care professionals.

Unlike some texts on sexuality and health, *Caring for Sexuality in Health and Illness* gives explicit acknowledgement to the difficulties that are experienced by practitioners in this field, and thought to the practical needs of managers and teachers looking to support them. Such recognition is important in its own right, but particularly germane at a time of significant staff shortages in the health services, and poor rates of staff retention. Many practitioners are aware of the ways in which the health of a patient or client may be compromised by psychosexual anxieties but are afraid to intervene in case they make matters worse. Others may be courageous enough to provide opportunities for their patients to raise concerns, but find working in this area highly challenging, and at times deeply painful. The book is helpful here at a number of levels. It offers a theoretical understanding of psychological development and psychosexual issues across the life cycle, and it counterbalances this through case examples which provide insights into, and opportunities to reflect on, the unique meanings and responses arising from individual experience. At the same time, taking a Balint approach means that the book's authors do not minimize or ignore the discomfort or disappointments experienced by practitioners. Instead, they argue for a form of clinical supervision that facilitates reflection on these experiences and promote a form of peer support that is constructive and developmental.

One other important feature of this book is its interactive nature, which takes a number of forms. Mirroring the Balint tradition, many of the case examples provided do not simply illustrate the text, but involve the reader at an experiential level through prompting an emotional as much as an intellectual response. There are also exercises to help the reader reflect on the issues raised in the text and relate them to their own area of practice. Perhaps most strikingly though, the book is offered as a springboard for future discussion: beyond the experience and wisdom to be found within these pages, there is the opportunity for readers to engage with the book's authors and to shape future seminars, workshops and publications on this important area.

This openness to future dialogue and to new ways of working is consistent with the work of Balint. However, it also reflects the tremendous enthusiasm and commitment on the part of the authors to make this kind of approach available to, and appropriate for, an increasing number and range of practitioners. This overall project, of which *Caring for Sexuality in Health and Illness* is an important and central element, represents a very special and exciting opportunity for health care practitioners who wish to develop their skills in sexual health care. It deserves every success.

Jan Savage, 2000

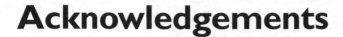

Acknowledgements

We would like to pay tribute to the many patients and seminar members who have taught us so much.

DW, DC, MR, JW 2000

Introduction

Diane Wells

BACKGROUND

The three authors of this book, Doreen Clifford, Marjorie Rutter and Jane Selby have worked together since the mid 1970s. Doreen Clifford led one of the three experimental Balint seminars (Balint 1957, Balint & Norell 1973) funded by the Department of Health for family planning nurses from 1974 to 1976; these were successful, so she continued. Jane and Marjorie, both family planning nurses, joined this second series. Since then, Balint groups for psychosexual practitioners have continued and diversified into Basic and Advanced Groups for practitioners, and Leaders' Groups. Currently these are conducted in Central and West London, Hertfordshire and Cornwall. Groups and workshops are usually set up in response to requests. The Association of Psychosexual Nurses offers a study day twice a year (see Appendix).

Jane has worked as a family planning practitioner for 37 years. Whilst working as a clinical teacher she ran the Principles of Psychosexual Counselling Course (approved by Joint Board of Clinical Nursing Studies, later English National Board for Nurses, Midwives and Health Visitors), in London from 1981 to 1990 (Randall 1992). She has conducted Balint seminars and workshops for both practitioners and leaders. Currently she is a nurse counsellor in psychosexual care (Selby 1997) for Camden and Islington Community Health Authority and leads seminars for midwives in Cornwall.

Marjorie started her work as a family planning practitioner in 1966. Together with Jane she taught on the psychosexual counselling course (ENB 985) for 10 years. Currently she is a specialist family planning practitioner and a counsellor for an assisted conception unit. She has a particular interest in the dynamics of psychological development and its relevance for clinical practice (Rutter & Rutter 1993).

Doreen has practised as a community midwife and a psychosocial nurse. Her group skills were honed at the Cassel Hospital (a therapeutic community in Surrey), as a clinical nurse and then as matron for 10 years. Since the mid-1970s she has been conducting Balint seminars in psychosexual care for both practitioners (Clifford 1998) and leaders.

Balint seminars are a method of reflecting on any practice that has an inter-personal element. Practitioners bring examples of their work with patients for discussion and scrutiny by a group of peers. Like all reflection the practitioner's wish to examine a piece of work often starts with a feeling of discomfort. Balint's particular contribution to this was to show how the feelings of the practitioner often emanate from the patient's world. Balint was a psychoanalyst who, like Freud (1973, orig. 1915–1917), thought there were features of psychoanalytic theory that could help in the understanding of everyday life. The Balint approach is discussed in Section 3. An account of Balint's work, and the use of his seminar method for both psychosexual and psychosocial care, is in the Appendix.

As the requests to run groups, conduct workshops and speak at conferences have been increasing, it seems clear that a book is required also. The authors asked me to help. My interest in Balint seminars, to study relationships in care, started when I joined the tutors' group, led by Doreen, at the Cassel Hospital in the early 1970s. Then, when employed there as a nurse and later a tutor, I worked with Doreen in education and training. Since then I have endeavoured to use a Balint approach within all my teaching (Wells 1998).

Before writing this book Doreen conducted extensive research using discussion groups and questionnaires to find out what practitioners, managers and teachers wanted. The results confirmed the impressions gained in earlier workshops and conferences. There was a thirst for something to help practi-tioners develop their skills. Readers are therefore encouraged to make links with their own practice whether as a clinical practitioner or a teacher. Many case studies and exercises are given to help in the development of skills. The book is not offered as a replacement for seminars and workshops. We hope it will be a stimulus and adjunct to training, helping practitioners to know about their existing skills, augmenting this with theoretical understanding and encouraging practitioners to experiment with new ways of working. The support for such exploration may come partly from this text, but it is also important to feel supported by peers and managers. This is discussed again at the end of this introduction, and in Sections 1 and 3.

Awareness, discomfort and their benefits

Many practitioners in health care are asking, 'How do I attend to the sexual health needs of patients?' There is an awareness that sexuality is often omitted from the care plan and the care given. This awareness may be associated with memories of specific patients who aroused in the practitioner feelings of wanting to do more, but not knowing quite what this might be, or how it could be achieved. Such awareness of unmet need is a crucial step towards developing skills to meet these needs. Authors of reflective practice, for example Schon (1987), Boud et al (1985) and de Lambert (1998), have all talked about the feeling of discomfort that often stimulates experiential learning. This book is written to respond to that discomfort, and to aid a process of learning that capitalises on the discomfort, by viewing it as a key to understanding the needs of patients. When a practitioner is aware of her own feelings she is often able to attune herself to her patients' feelings, and so begin the study of emotional experience and relationships that will form the basis of understanding patients' needs.

There are other practitioners who say, 'I think this work of sexual care is for specialists – counsellors maybe. It's not really part of my work as a practitioner in health care.' We all have spheres of work about which we are less certain, and in which we are perhaps less skilled. It is often argued that teamwork can ensure that clients' needs are met with competent practice. The idea is that if practitioner A is not very good at this sort of care, probably practitioner B or C can step in. If, however, sexual care is not acknowledged as part of every health care practitioner's concern and responsibility, then the principle of holistic care is lost, and patients may lose out too.

The sexual health care discussed in this book relates to the implicit and explicit requests made to practitioners in the midst of everyday work. The request for a physical examination, or when a patient asks, 'Will I be alright?', or 'What about when I go home to my partner?' are sometimes ways of patients thinking out loud about a concern. If the practitioner is able to offer a 'bridge for safe crossing' (see Chapter 1) then the concern can be explored. When this happens, patient and practitioner often acknowledge the value of discussing it *then*. It seems the moment is right and there is a need to catch this moment.

Making care visible to practitioners

Feeling uncertain about one's skills in sexual care does not necessarily mean that the health care practitioner is devoid of skills. When observed, those who protest their ignorance in sexual care might demonstrate considerable skill. The care may be given intuitively, and be highly valued by the patient. However, if the care remains at this level, that is, not expressed in words, it has a secret quality, known only to the practitioner and client in the moment of care. Sometimes this intuitive care is not valued by practitioners, and often it is not remembered by them. The reason for this seems to be associated with a sense of humility on the part of the practitioner, but also there may be a fear that increased awareness and thinking about feelings will destroy the 'natural' empathy and much valued 'intuition'. We hope this book will help to make intuitive, invisible care much more visible. This is not just for advertisement, or for political ends (status, power, money), but rather to allow for further development of practice.

There is a need for practitioners to make care visible to themselves, so that they can understand the elements of their care and develop their skills. If practitioners are going to develop skills through awareness of feelings and the study of relationships, then these experiences have to be thought about. Thinking about feelings is very beneficial, and in our experience the result is more sensitive and skilled care.

Identity and sexuality

Being close to and knowing about the sexuality of patients may seem like stepping into unknown territory. Yet as practitioners help, touch, educate, support and talk and listen to their patients, the interactions are likely to involve the patient's sense of identity. This sense of self or identity is not asexual but includes the sexual self. A practitioner may listen to a client's story of, for example, a life-cycle change about growing up or growing older, or about illness or bereavement. Such stories are likely to be concerned with the changing sense of self and identity and we would argue that this identity includes sexual identity. The practitioner's response is important because it may help or impede the sense of sexual identity.

Health care is usually given at a time of change, e.g. changes related to:

1. emotional growth and development across the life span
2. illness
3. psychosocial events such as changes in relationships.

At these times identities, and that means sexual identities, are developing and are in a process of change. Bury's (1988) work demonstrates how the onset of illness changes relationships which then have to be renegotiated. He points out that illness is a social event. Similarly it could be argued that life-cycle changes (e.g. growing up or growing older) and psychosocial events such as marriage, divorce and bereavement all necessitate changes in close relationships, and usually a change in the sense of identity. Since we are sexual beings, our relationships and identities include our sense of our own sexuality. Practitioners of health care are working in the midst of these very processes of change and development, hence with their patients' changing sense of themselves as (sexual) people. We hope this book will help to remove the brackets from the practice. The fear of stepping into the unknown seems therefore to be a fear of realising where one is.

THE BOOK AS A LEARNING TEXT

A text cannot 'provide learning' since the learning required to practise is much more complex than information to be gained. It is hard to imagine any use for learning that is simply repetition of stored information. Nevertheless the complexity of learning and development of skills useful for practice are issues not always addressed in books. We hope that this text will be perceived as one offering active learning opportunities. Case examples are used throughout the book. In Sections 1 and 3 the reader is encouraged to reflect on the examples, to undertake exercises and to collect their own examples for reflection.

Three sections of the book

1. Developing psychosexual awareness
2. Life span emotional development and sexuality
3. Coaching for psychosexual awareness.

This perhaps unusual arrangement, starting with practice and then proceeding to theory, has been chosen because we believe that the theoretical understanding of psychosexual care is derived from the understanding of people, not the other way around. Therefore the experience of practice is the first area for study. The final section is devoted to coaching the practitioner – using Balint-style (Balint et al 1993, Main 1989) seminars. The term 'coach' is taken from the writing of Schon (1987) since it fits well with the principles of Balint seminars. 'The coach tries to discern what the student understands, what her peculiar difficulties are about, (and) what she already knows how to do ...' (Schon 1987, p 101).

Each of the sections both illuminates and relies upon the other two. Sections 1 and 2 might be particularly appropriate for practitioners, whereas Sections 2 and 3 might be particularly valuable for trainers, but practitioners often find they are also the coaches, and teachers and trainers will find in Section 1 many examples and exercises for use in discussion or workshops.

In the first section much of the material has been gathered from practitioners and demonstrates the sort of work possible. Some of the examples have been described and discussed in Balint psychosexual seminars (see Section 3) and so the discussion demonstrates how the practitioner can be in tune with her patients' feelings, although this may be difficult and all practitioners have failures as well as successes. Doreen (like Jane in Section 3) shows that whatever happens between patient and practitioner it is all deemed worthy of study at the next seminar. The examples are also used as a basis for study, and exercises are suggested to help the reader make explorations and application of the ideas.

The second section is concerned with psychological development across the life span, with particular reference to psychosexual issues. Two interacting facets of development are clarified: first, the complex interplay of genes, environment and biological maturation, and second, the unique meaning given to an experience. These dynamics of psychological development are illuminated with research findings, discussion and a range of case studies.

The third section is written particularly with group leaders in mind. Leaders may be lecturers, trainers, senior staff, or one of a peer group who is convening a study group. Jane discusses the features of group work, indicating what the leader might experience. She suggests ways in which the leader may both negotiate situations and develop skills through the experience. Balint (1957) training seminars are discussed as a mode of reflection, supervision and action research. The difference between this and other forms of reflection is the use of the practitioner's feelings to understand the patient's world.

It is recommended that leaders do not work alone in this role, but seek training to support and develop the work. Anyone who has experience of working in face to face groups where discussion is the method of work will know how important it is to have ongoing training and support. The leader is otherwise in a very vulnerable position, and the work of the group may well be impeded or even stopped. In our experience, leaders need courage to start this work, and then need training to use this courage for further work.

LOOKING TO THE FUTURE

We do not regard any of this as the final word but rather offer it as some ideas from experiences in psychosexual work and training. We hope that the examples, discussions and exercises will stimulate many readers to take up this work in diverse ways, to continue the learning and discourse. We look forward to meeting as many readers as possible as a result of this book. We plan to run workshops based around the ideas here and in response to readers' comments and suggestions. At the back of the book you will find a response sheet which you might like to photocopy, fill in and return. In that way, future work in seminars, workshops and books is more likely to fit with practitioner requirements.

One final note, throughout the book both the practitioner and the developing person are referred to as 'she'. The majority of health care practitioners are women, but we hope the men reading this book do not feel excluded.

REFERENCES

Balint M 1957 The doctor, his patient and the illness. Pitman Medical, London

Balint E, Norell J S (eds) 1973 Six minutes for the patient. Tavistock, London

Balint E, Courtenay M, Elder A, Hull S, Julian P 1993 The doctor, the patient and the group. Routledge, London

Boud D, Keogh R, Walker D 1985 Reflection: turning experience into learning. Kogan Page, London

Bury M 1988 Meanings at risk: the experience of arthritis. In: Anderson R, Bury M (eds) Living with chronic illness. Unwin Hyman, London

Clifford D 1998 Psychosexual nursing seminars. In: Barnes E, Griffiths P, Ord J, Wells D (eds) 1998 Face to face with distress. Butterworth Heinemann, Oxford

de Lambert L 1998 Learning through experience. In: Barnes E, Griffiths P, Ord J, Wells D (eds) 1998 Face to face with distress. Butterworth Heinemann, Oxford

Freud S 1973 Sigmund Freud 1. Introductory lectures on psychoanalysis. Penguin, Middlesex

Main T 1989 Training for the acquisition of knowledge or the development of skill? In: Johns J (ed) The ailment and other psychoanalytic essays. Free Association Books, London

Randall E 1992 Preparation for psychosexual nursing: results of survey of ENB 985 at the Olive Haydon School of Midwifery-Lewisham Hospital. Goldsmiths College, London

Rutter M, Rutter M 1993 Developing minds: challenge and continuity across the lifespan. Penguin, Middlesex

Schon D A 1987 Educating the reflective practitioner. Jossey Bass, San Francisco

Selby J 1997 Psychosexual and emotional care. In: Andrews G (ed) Women's sexual health. Baillière Tindall, London

Wells D 1998 Biographical work with older people. In: Barnes E, Griffiths P, Ord J, Wells D (eds) Face to face with distress. Butterworth Heinemann, Oxford

Section 1

Developing psychosexual awareness

1

Psychosexual awareness in health care

Doreen Clifford

KEY ISSUES

- ◆ Managing the boundaries.
- ◆ Disturbances to sexuality in health and illness
- ◆ The professional use of self
- ◆ Linking practice and the page

INTRODUCTION

This section of the book deals with the issue of how health care professionals manage the boundary between personal involvement and professional detachment, particularly when faced by people in distress. We all have needs and vulnerabilities. Sometimes feelings of shame and fragility affect us when the personal places of our lives are troubled. From this recognition in ourselves comes the opportunity to grow skills, such as being aware of and responding to painful feelings expressed by people who seek our professional help.

Section 1 will explore those areas of feeling within the practitioner, which when acknowledged can help us to understand the therapeutic potential in the professional–patient relationship. The practitioner is involved in a process of remembering and recounting, not just what happened with the patient, but also what it felt like – a process that is often difficult. As Butterworth & Faugier (1992) suggest, practitioners are rarely asked to explore and explain their practice, although with clinical supervision there is more opportunity for such activities.

How then do we respond to needs that may be expressed by a look or a gesture? Many practitioners who have contributed to this book use the image of 'building a bridge for patients to cross in safety' (Clifford 1998), a phrase that will be explained in Chapter 2. Difficult feelings and ideas can then be expressed more readily in words. The image of the bridge is used to convey that an offer is being made, but there is no obligation. This is very important since it protects the patient's right to privacy.

The paradox of involvement and detachment in the professional management of boundaries is described by de Raeve (1998) who says, 'engagement may be important but so also is the maintenance of a degree of distance and objectivity, which is essential for both (professional) and patient in order for (care) to occur.' She goes on to emphasise that boundaries must be drawn to protect the privacy of the patient and the health care professional and permit the survival of the professional encounter. This subject is developed further in Chapter 6.

BECOMING AWARE OF THE BODY IN HEALTH

In good health, we remain for the most part unaware of our body and its functions; we take ourselves for granted. Walking, for example, is unremarkable unless we become out of breath, or a knee or ankle gives a twinge of pain. Then we notice that our body, which usually follows the commands of the nervous system to walk or breathe without our taking conscious thought, suddenly requires us to take notice. When we are well, our breathing is unremarked by us and we need take little notice that minute by minute we are sustained by it.

Try an experiment: count the number of breaths you take in a minute; the very taking-thought, the interruption to natural control, will probably disrupt the regular pattern of your breathing. It is when the functions of our body are disturbed that we become conscious of the normal and are awakened to the broken flow of the unconscious control we exercise over ourselves.

The private nature of sexuality

As illustrated above for breathing and other bodily functions, so it is with sexual health. Taken for granted by most people most of the time, if its functions, or feelings about functions, become disrupted, sensitivities are wakened to distress in body and mind.

Sexuality is a personal and private part of life for most people. There is a proper 'shyness', which requires respect by both health professional and patient. Nevertheless, it can be argued that the professional responsibility is to try to be aware that feelings about sexuality, often unspoken, can influence health, complicate responses to treatment and even impair recovery.

What happened here?

The case study below is a story of a patient, meeting with a nurse, where feelings got in the way of them both dealing with a problem.

Case study 1.1

A healthy woman in early middle age had grown increasingly concerned about small, hard, white nodules on her vulva. She attended her local practice for a routine cervical smear with a practice nurse she liked. She hoped at the same time to speak about her concern. Despite feeling shy, she was determined to mention the problem. However, the smear was taken and the woman went home; neither she nor the nurse had addressed the fact of the vulval changes. The woman was too shy – and the nurse? Why did she not talk to the woman about something so obvious?

We might wonder why was it so difficult for the nurse to work with this matter, to say, 'I see you have some small hard areas here, do they worry you?' Perhaps the nurse thought she needed to know what they were or what to do. Was there a way she might have opened a discussion with the patient?

Perhaps the difficulty was of a different nature. Was she in fact so sensitive to the patient's unspoken inhibitions, which had prevented her from speaking about her labia, that the nurse lost touch with her professional expertise? She in turn, perhaps, became inhibited about the personal nature of the visit.

The nurse could have referred the client on after some discussion, if it seemed suitable. Instead, the patient left feeling frustrated with herself, embarrassed, neglected and guilty about her unspoken criticism of a nurse whom she had previously trusted.

How might we understand this disappointing meeting? In studying the patient's story, two feelings are apparent:

◆ Her anxiety
◆ Her embarrassment.

We might be tempted to consider that if the nodules were on the woman's arm, her breast, or even on the inner aspect of her upper thigh, she would have managed to draw attention to them. But, they were on her labia. (Section 2 of the book contains some interesting reading about how we come to own and view our genitals.)

The nurse was also faced with several difficulties:

◆ Years of training and experience may have led her to believe that she was responsible for recognising whatever symptoms were present.

◆ Perhaps she did not recognise the nodules and thus retreated from acknowledging them.
◆ The unspoken anxiety from the woman of which she must have been, at least unconsciously, aware and which seemed unspeakable to them both.

Noticeably, there was no problem for either woman in taking the cervical smear, but it was the labial nodules that were avoided. We can only guess at what happened in the professional–patient relationship. Was the nurse flooded by the patient's embarrassment or was it her professional sense of self that was paralysed? We shall never know, but we do know that the patient's difficulty received no attention.

Other opportunities for practitioners

After discussion, nurses sometimes see alternative ways of responding to such difficulties. In a seminar group, for example, the nurse in the example above could safely reflect with colleagues about the occasion and the feelings aroused in her. From this discussion she might, for example, have considered appropriate ways to contact the patient again. (See Section 2 for descriptions of psychosexual seminars.)

Disturbances to whole body sexuality

It would be a mistake to see sexuality as only related to genitourinary areas of the body. What about someone with a facial injury? How do they see themselves, how is their image of themselves changed and with what result for their current or future relationships? How might their partner feel about them now? What about the loss of a limb? How might that change a person's perceptions of themselves or the attitudes of a partner? What are the fears of returning to a sexual relationship after such a change? The irritating nature of skin lesions does not just irritate the skin but the whole person. How might their partner perceive living with them? Losing a breast, an eye, a kidney, teeth even, what difference might that make? Coping with stoma care is about more than competence and cleanliness. What of the changes to the body and one's personal odour? The threat of death that a diagnosis of cancer conveys can also impinge into the depth of a close relationship in many ways. Bereavement, for some people, may take several years to resolve allowing for the possibility of a new relationship, whilst for others, a fresh partnership is possible much sooner and for some, never. Parkes & Markus (1998) suggest that though the grief that follows physical losses is different from the grief that follows loss of a person, there are important similarities. In sexual health care, the practitioner needs to grow a particular sensitivity to the understanding of the closeness of these two kinds of grief.

Disturbances to sexuality in health

Not all psychosexual issues are related to illness. Other life events, such as childbirth, may give rise to feelings about changes in the body. Along with the delights of a new baby may be worries about what happened 'down there'. Is there damage, stretching, splitting, will it ever be the same again? What effect will the stitches have, what will they do to me, is there any space left for entry of a penis? What happens to the caring partner who witnessed the delivery? No matter how well prepared, what did he experience and what are his fantasies for the future of their sexual relationship? Milk smells and can make clothes wet and breasts larger and tender – what is the effect on the sexual relationship? Not to mention the baby, the new member who has demands of his own to make known to the family group, especially at night in that time the couple previously had for themselves.

And losses of a variety of kinds? Loss of a baby, loss of a pregnancy, a choice to terminate a pregnancy. What may the outcomes of these be and what feelings may be aroused by them?

All of us are sexual beings. Our sexuality is an integral part of us, we have no choice. It is there before birth and until our death; it is both more and less than gender. Skrine (1997) writes of the intertwined nature of bodily and emotional pains; Section 1 makes a plea for health care professionals to recognise this fact by increasing their skills for responding to patients who seek help with sexual unhappiness.

THE TASK OF RECOGNITION

The health care professional caring for patients' sexuality has a role in recognising the presence of sexuality in every part of their work, to look for it in both health and illness. There is a need for both recognition and help with the feelings of people whose lives are disordered by acute illness, hospitalisation, surgery and chronic ill-health. Many workers already have skills enabling them to work alongside patients in caring for sexuality. Sometimes these skills remain dormant or are unrecognised for what they are, namely the ability to respond to human pain. The advent of HIV and AIDS has meant that advanced skills of listening and counselling have been developed by practitioners in this work who have much to offer other health care workers about responding to the individual patients' psychosexual needs.

Difficulties of responding

The complexity of the role of the health care professional is such that patients' sexual feelings may be avoided. Reasons given for not being able to recognise and respond to psychosexual needs are listed in Box 1.1. The reasons are all valid, and yet many professional people would like to offer help, but feel themselves at a loss to know how.

Developing approaches to patients

The delicate balance in maintaining the boundaries of public and private, involvement and detachment can be helped by reflective practice, supervision and further training. Consideration of 'building emotional bridges' between practitioner and patient forms the basis for this section of the book. With time and continuing training, sensitive health care professionals can develop their awareness of patients' needs, and appreciate those issues, either spoken or unspoken, that are important to patients.

THE PROFESSIONAL USE OF SELF

The term 'professional use of self' is used frequently in this book, as a way of expressing the practitioner's use of their own individuality whilst relating to a patient in a professional way; that is, how a health care practitioner manages the boundary between personal involvement and professional detachment, particularly when faced by people in distress. This boundary, a fine line between distance and closeness, is explored in some detail in Chapter 6.

The friendly, approachable way a confident practitioner relates to someone who is a patient offers a co-equal partnership in care. The practitioner–patient relationship allows for patients to move easily between the different parts

---

Box 1.1 Reasons given for avoiding patients' sexual feelings

◆ Time
◆ Pressure of work
◆ Not knowing enough
◆ Feeling uneasy
◆ Not wishing to cause offence
◆ Shyness
◆ Not being at ease
◆ Not feeling responsible
◆ Not having the words
◆ Inhibitions
◆ Lack of privacy.

of themselves that may be experienced during the course of illness and treatment. For example, someone who is severely ill may be more in touch with their child-like, even baby-like self at times, perhaps when requiring toiletting or intimate bodily care. This does not mean that they are regarded as a baby, but as an adult requiring the same asexual attentions to their body as an infant does. Likewise, when patient and practitioner together are exploring psychosexual disturbances during treatment, the practitioner is able to maintain the partnership – as a partner alongside the patient trying to understand the difficulties being experienced. The professional use of self allows movement between these two and numerous other kinds of attention and maintains both the practitioner and the patient as intact functioning adults.

The relationship is not friendship, but rather the use of the practitioner's self to maintain closeness and a perception of herself and the other, who in this instance is a patient or client.

SHARED TASKS INVOLVED WHEN USING THIS BOOK

Reading a book to aid one's thinking about practice is most useful when recognised as a shared task between the reader and the writing. This discourse makes for a discussion in which the reader plays a vital part. It is the reader's practice alongside which the words on the page should be set, measured, assessed and considered (Box 1.2).

Box 1.2 Questions for readers to ask while reading

◆ Do I agree with this statement?

◆ Does this make sense to me?

◆ Do I recognise this issue occurring in my own practice?

◆ Is the situation described one with which I am familiar?

◆ Might I understand yesterday's clinical encounter in this new light?

◆ Does that point of view help my thinking and the development of my own sexual health care practice?

The task of considering and assessing fresh ideas and their application to the reader's practice is vital when using this book. Interpersonal skills cannot be learned from the printed page but reading can provide a basis for discussion with colleagues to reflect together upon possible application to your own developing sexual health care practice. Bion (1975) wrote, 'the time we have is limited, so we must learn to read people.'

CONCLUSION

Psychosexual care, i.e. holistic care of body and mind, requires continuing training to ease its integration into our everyday work. You will be invited to reflect upon the feelings you experience in your encounters with patients and to consider how this awareness can help in the development of your skills. There are reflection points for discussion and exercises to use; on your own, with another interested person, or in groups. You are encouraged to keep a reflective diary. Most of all we hope you will find this book an interactive opportunity to aid you in integrating sensitive sexual care into your own practice.

REFERENCES

Bion W R 1975 Brazilian lectures 2. Imago Editoria, Rio de Janeiro
Butterworth T, Faugier J 1992 The supervisory relationship. In: Clinical supervision and mentorship in nursing. Stanley Thomas, London, pp 4–5
Clifford D 1998 Psychosexual awareness in everyday nursing. Nursing Standard 12: 39, 42–45
de Raeve L 1998 Knowing the patient: how much and how well? In: Barnes E, Griffiths P et al (eds) Face to face with distress. Butterworth Heinemann, Oxford
Parkes C M, Markus A (eds) 1998 Coping with loss. BMA Books, London
Skrine R 1997 Blocks and freedoms in sexual life. Radcliffe Medical, Oxford

2

Professional awareness in psychosexual care
Struggling to understand

Doreen Clifford

KEY ISSUES

◆ Recognising patient's wishes for help
◆ Psychosomatic care
◆ The feelings of the health care worker
◆ Developing skills through recognizing feelings

INTRODUCTION

The struggle to understand is a constant in the work of caring for people. It is always within a particular relationship that the value of the professional use of self is recognised (see Chapter 1). Each person's individuality means that the health care practitioner is constantly learning, developing and adjusting their sensitivity to understanding each patient. This chapter will discuss how a practitioner develops her skills.

Psychosexual skills in a scientific world

It is recognised that professional skills and knowledge need to be developed throughout the practitioner's working life as underlined by the PREPP programme (Post Registration Education and Practice Project) (UKCC 1990). However, finding a way of developing knowledge and skills that are meaningful for the practitioner is often difficult. Those working face to face with clients require a range of psychosocial skills, but much of the Western education system values knowledge at the expense of skills, and values cognitive skills rather than emotional skills.

There is a professional balance we need to keep between the recognition of science as the way forward and the knowledge that unresolved feelings can impede recovery. Holloway (1997) suggests that:

Scientific thinking and the life of the intellect seem so often to be the working goal of the professions. Many people work so hard with their intellect that their feelings are neglected, neither respected nor alerted ...the area of the mind we call feelings has come to be seen as doubtful and of little value in the professional sphere.

We may recognise this view but, by increasing skills in psychosexual awareness and care, we challenge this assumption that feelings are unimportant.

Recognising patients' wishes for help

Sometimes, the hope left at the bottom of Pandora's box for the patient, when all the demons have flown, is the response of the professional health care worker who dares to ask 'what did it feel like for you?' or 'is there anything more you want to talk about?'

A number of studies indicate that patients are often seeking more than they are offered (Waterhouse & Metcalfe 1991). Snow (1994) points out to physiotherapists how the sexual health of patients is an important part of their recovery from physical symptoms. She describes how the technique of improved listening has led to a heightened awareness and better interpretation of feelings which patients may have been fearful of expressing. She makes the telling point that this technique as an integral part of patient care does not necessarily extend the time allotted to treatment.

As mentioned in the introduction, psychosexual awareness is the integration into one's practice of the facts of human sexuality and its vulnerability. The skill is to learn to balance this aspect of the person alongside the multiplicity of other necessary clinical data that we need to make clinical decisions. As in all holistic care, it is the maintenance of this balance of the physical and the psychological, the psychosomatic, mind and body, which is the goal for high quality practice. Human sexuality is part of this body–mind continuum.

Sexuality is also a personal and private part of life for most people. Privacy belongs here, to be respected by both health care worker and patient. It is important to be aware that feelings about sexuality are often disturbed by treatment. Fears and anxieties, although often unspoken, can influence and complicate responses to treatment and even impair recovery.

Thinking about psychosomatic care

Psychosomatic means that the psyche and the soma are so intertwined that changes in one cause change in the other. When feelings are disturbed, bodily functions are liable to be disturbed also. Similarly, changes in the body bring about changes in feelings. This being so, it is not appropriate for care to be focused exclusively on either the body or the mind. Care needs to focus on the whole person. Psychosomatic understanding is necessary for holistic care. Psychosexual care links this understanding to sexual health where our awareness of the body–mind links are so important.

Health, illness and the part feelings have to play

Case study 2.1

Mrs M who had, some 20 years before, been successfully treated for an auto-immune response disease talked to her GP. She told him that she had symptoms which led her to believe that she was experiencing a recurrence. He examined her and told her that it was unlikely. On several further occasions she mentioned this matter; he continued to reassure her. She became increasingly tired and unwell. She felt the doctor did not believe her and was not taking her seriously. Her family encouraged her to return and eventually she did so. This time she made a firm request for re-referral to the original treating institution. Although indicating his doubtfulness, the GP agreed. At her first consultation with the specialist she was treated seriously. A full history was taken, she was examined and a series of tests was organised. She says she left full of gratitude at the way she was received and believed, and she felt 'on a high'.

The interesting feature was the response of this woman. She tells how, for the first time in months, her tiredness decreased. Her symptoms remained but she ceased to worry about them, feeling they would receive appropriate treatment. She felt better in herself.

Mrs M's story is an example of the mind–body link; think about about how and why things happen. There are powerful implications for professional practice when engaging with psychosomatic care and recognising the indivisibility of mind and body.

Why did Mrs M feel so much better following the specialist consultation? How might we understand what happened? Are there any implications for your own practice?

The busy GP had done his best but we notice that Mrs M kept returning to the surgery. We observe that time is taken in repeated consultations, yet neither doctor nor patient are satisfied. Could it have been her sense of helplessness and repressed anger at not being taken seriously that provoked Mrs M to feel so tired? Note that she was referred to the place of her choice when she made a specific straightforward request. That is, when *she* took *responsibility* for firmly requesting further help. The GP responded differently when she moved from being a 'good' patient who was quiet and compliant, to being an adult with a mind of her own (Sadgrove 1997). The result was a consultation with a specialist in her illness. Then, with symptoms still present, she was less tired and felt better. Why was this?

You may find it useful to reflect upon Mrs M's story of the psyche and the soma either alone or in discussion with colleagues. What, if anything, does this story suggest to you about the psychosomatic implications for care in your practice? How do you listen and respond to what a patient says to you so that both of you understand what kind of help the patient wants? Do you have any examples from your recent practice?

There is interesting further reading in Broom (1997), a doctor working in Christchurch, New Zealand. He believes that most illness may be understood as the body showing what is happening to the patient emotionally. If bodies are treated separately from feelings; the 'dualism' of Western culture is perpetuated. Alternatively, practitioners can challenge this through practising holistic care.

Reflection point 2.1

Please make some notes on your reflections about the above example. You may like to comment upon the changes in the GP–patient relationship and the way it moved between detachment and engagement.

Some interesting questions are:

◆ Why did the GP, apparently, not believe that the patient felt ill?

◆ Why did Mrs M allow herself to feel so tired and ill before returning to the surgery to make her wishes clear to the GP?

◆ It was the same GP, but why did he respond to her positively on the final occasion?

◆ Which part of Mrs M was preventing her adult self from taking charge?

◆ Why did she feel so much better after the physician saw her?

◆ Was there something else in her life that her body was reflecting?

Sexual care in health

Professional clinical work requires another balance to be maintained, that of managing and caring for health as well as illness. When working with healthy people, practitioners may be alerted to disturbances in sexual health by word or demeanour. Courage may be required of the practitioner to test her perceptions of whether this is a request for help that should be followed through.

Who are the healthy people we see in our everyday practice? Some are the people that we see as part of daily working practice (Box 2.1).

Healthy people may be seeking help in more ways than their presentation suggests. Holistic care requires that we understand and accept the indivisibility of self if psychosexuality is to be integrated into practice. We may begin in simple ways. Some physiotherapists, for example, make it their practice to suggest that partners could be helpfully involved in treatment. In massaging injured limbs or helping with exercise regimes it may be possible for a couple to become closer. The understanding of the physiotherapist that touching can not only aid healing but may also draw a couple together at times of pain or injury has helped many people. Physical sharing may also lead to sharing talk about feelings and opportunities to explore other shared experiences.

Working with feelings in health

Pregnancy and childbirth may disrupt lives. ('Relate' suggest that childbirth is the most frequent trigger to marital breakdown.) Feelings about what happened need attention if full health is to be regained after these events.

The gratitude so many people express to practitioners after their hospitalisation should not be taken at face value. Conversations with patients and their families about how they experienced what professionals perceive as routine procedures may reveal hidden distress.

Box 2.1 Examples of healthy patients

◆ people, mostly young, presenting with sports injuries to be cared for by physiotherapists

◆ young families in the community seen by the health visitor

◆ elderly couples coming to the practice nurse, perhaps for flu jabs

◆ people with disabilities seen by many practitioners

◆ women of all ages presenting for routine cervical smears in family planning consultations

◆ men attending well man clinics or the GP practice for health checks

◆ men and women of all ages, who are seeking contraceptive advice

◆ women seeking termination of pregnancy

◆ couples seeking advice on conception.

Many health care workers recognise this distress alongside the need for clinical action. Following their clinical action during the management of labour and delivery, some midwives make it their business to spend time with newly delivered couples, and offer an opportunity for them to talk over and think about their experience of childbirth. A skilled midwife may be able to help a couple to feel comfortable enough to discuss what may have been, for them, two very different experiences of the labour and delivery (see case study below).

Case study 2.2

In a psychosexual workshop, a midwife spoke of one such occasion. After a long delivery, a healthy baby was born. The parents seemed happy but exhausted and the husband returned home for a rest. On his return the midwife saw him sitting alone, waiting for his wife to wake. When asked how he was, he explained how distressed he had felt by the delivery. He told how, on going home, he had gone into a deep sleep and woke to find that he had wet the bed. He was shocked, but he seemed to be acknowledging the tumult of feeling in himself, so delighted at being a father, so happy with the baby and also so distressed at the pain he had witnessed at his wife's delivery of this baby. He had felt so helpless, he said. As he told this he looked relieved. He thanked the midwife for listening to him, especially as now he was ready to share with his wife both what had distressed and delighted him.

What we may observe from this story are the risks taken by these two people; the midwife in offering to listen and the man by telling her of his experiences. She, by listening carefully and in silence and he, in daring to show his feelings, demonstrate just what unexpected exchanges can happen when professionals are trusted and become brave enough to listen, without needing to 'make it better'.

Sexual health requires professionals to be alert to patients' expressed and unexpressed needs. The expertise required is that of listening with close attention to the feelings being expressed. To do this, however, we need to take risks (see also Chapter 4, Making space for new ideas). One of these risks is in letting go of 'knowing'. The skill to be developed is of respecting what we hear, however uncomfortable. We do not have to agree with other people's feelings to understand their pain. Actively listening and accepting what is heard is necessary to understand what it was like.

The feelings of the health care worker

Our feelings may prove to be unexpected and may either free the health care worker to move to understanding and action, or provoke anxiety and professional paralysis.

We are free to choose, but it is not easy. Reflect on the two stories: the midwife who listened from the beginning, and the GP who eventually listened; both practitioners reached engagement with the client.

The midwife, in the example above, chose to listen to the man in distress following the birth. She apparently did nothing but respect his feelings and stay alongside his pain; she neither judged nor preached. We can admire the support she gave as potentially enabling this couple to return to psychosexual health together. His feelings had been shared and accepted by this professional woman and, we hope, with his partner. Consequently perhaps, they found themselves more ready to begin their new life together as parents.

Working with healthy relatives of ill people – partners, parents and families

As in the story above, caring for healthy functioning relatives may seem an unnecessary addition to the already overfull schedule of a practitioner. Who is to do the caring? What has this to do with psychosexual care? Surely it is enough to ask for us to develop our skills with named patients?

However, a major disruption for a healthy couple is likely to occur should a baby or child become seriously ill. Consider this statement and the following story of disruption in the life of a previously content couple.

Mr James is speaking of the life-threatening illness of his newly born first son, Edward.

Case study 2.3

'Angela, my wife, was in hospital with the baby, she had a small room adjoining the baby unit. I was at work all day, finding it difficult to concentrate and worrying all the time. I spent the evenings in the hospital so I became very tired and irritable. Weekends were worse. I was in hospital all the time where I felt unable to do anything useful. I did not know how to help either Angela or Edward. Angela, on the other hand, became good at helping the nurses and coping with the baby's illness. She was wonderful, I didn't know she would be able to do such things. I really admire her.'
He went on to say that he felt himself to be of no use in the situation.
The baby is now fully recovered and they have another small child.
Asked about the effect upon their relationship, he said, 'People expect it would have brought us closer together, but sadly, we are further apart now and cannot seem to get close anymore since the baby's illness.'

There is no doubt that this couple valued the opportunity to stay with and share the care of their sick infant. However, we can see from the father's story that this also disrupted the couple's valued marital relationship, as Mr James felt he had become isolated from his wife, Angela. We have no report from her but may guess that she experienced similar feelings. This sense of isolation in a relationship under strain is very painful. It is clear from the example above that these two adults continued to struggle with their relationship, maybe with their sexual lives too. This expression of his sadness by Mr James at the loss of their erstwhile closeness raises many issues for professionals.

Reflection point 2.2

◆ What do you think might have helped this couple at the time of their baby's illness?

◆ Do you think someone could have initiated a discussion between the couple to share what the experience for each of them was during their baby's illness?

◆ The people at hand were the health care professionals, themselves also caring for other sick infants and children on the ward. Who might appropriately have helped the couple and how?

◆ You might like to make a few notes as you reflect upon how you would like to approach a similar situation in your own practice.

◆ Do you foresee the likelihood of psychosexual difficulties at such a time? What then might be the most useful role of the professional?

Sexual care in illness

There is another choice for the practitioner, i.e. to avoid the care of sexuality and to stay with the known and safe way of working. At a meeting where a paper was given on sexual care in their specialty, some health care workers had made this other choice. They seemed offended when it was suggested that the seriously ill patients they care for might be helped by an opportunity to talk over how they see their illness affecting their sexual lives. One worker said, 'It is difficult enough to talk to my own lovely children about sex. How could I talk about it to a patient!' This perhaps demonstrates something of the confusion some workers have about psychosexual care in everyday working situations. Work with adults, however ill they may be, means offering them an opportunity to talk over their feelings with their key professional worker – not an expert in sexology, as some people fear they are being invited to become.

Sexual awareness with death and dying

The deaths of much loved partners

Mrs Eve's story below is an occasion when no help was required from professionals but is an account of the closeness of two people. Mr and Mrs Eve had lived through many years together in sickness and in health, and their story illustrates that human sexuality is not only confined to the act of intercourse. The intimacy of body closeness and the warmth of cuddling and bodily care can also be an expression of sexuality. Theirs is a story of closeness and longing, persisting even after death.

Case study 2.4

Mrs Eve, a lady in her 80s, had nursed her even older husband through his final years of ill health. He had become increasingly disabled by Parkinson's disease. Latterly he was incontinent, unable to feed himself and barely able to communicate with her verbally. They had community carers to help, but the hard work of the majority of his care was hers.

One night she woke up and found he had died quietly in bed beside her. She got up and washed him, changed his night clothes and, since it was still only 4.00 am, she returned to bed alongside him to sleep until morning.

Her elder sister asked why she hadn't sought help from the family, and was told there was no point waking anyone at that time of day. Anyway, they had slept together for all these years, so why not now when she wanted to be close to him for the last time?

Later Mrs Eve divided his ashes and half she scattered in the crematorium garden where many of their family lie. As a former seaman, his wish was for a burial at sea. The high cost of this was beyond her. But, respecting his wishes, she awaited the concurrence of a receding tide and an off-shore wind to scatter them in the sea close to their marital home.

You may consider that Mr Eve was fortunate to die at home alongside a life-long, loving partner who was able to make a special and fitting farewell to him in her own way. Sadly, there are other experiences. This extract from a letter draws to our attention a particular sense of unnecessary human pain experienced by a couple.

My partner died of cancer about 20 months ago, and I am vividly aware that health care, especially for the dying, seems to ignore sexual and intimacy needs. In hospitals and hospices, privacy between partners is virtually unachievable. Spenco mattresses for home care only get supplied in single bed sizes, so if you want to share a bed there is a 'cliff' between you.

Reflection point 2.3

In reflecting on the opportunities to care for the second couple, is there anything in your practice that might be changed to increase a sense of privacy? You might care to make some notes about this. Please pay especial attention to your own feelings. What does 'intimate' mean to you, for example?

Also, you could discuss these issues with your colleagues. Here are some questions you might like to set yourself; you can probably think of more.

◆ Do opportunities exist on your ward for a couple to have intimate moments together? It may be that the comfort of close cuddling would help. It might mean sharing a bed to be really close for a short while. Who might be troubled by this?

◆ Do you ever consider that a patient might be bathed by a partner and that this would provide an opportunity for intimate care in privacy?

◆ Are there opportunities for couples to hold hands and talk quietly together, without the rest of the room/ward knowing or overhearing?

◆ If you work in the community, have you ever considered drawing your manager's attention to the inadequacies of single mattresses?

◆ How do you feel about dying people and their partners having sexual needs?

◆ Have you ever discussed these issues with a couple?

Developing skills through feelings

Awareness of sexuality during everyday work

The work described next was undertaken by an experienced and skilled practitioner. We are able to benefit from her experience because she was brave enough to describe how she felt. In this situation her feelings got in the way of her offering the help her patient probably needed. The example below shows how complex this work is.

The patient is a healthy woman receiving routine sexual health care. In the first instance the practitioner paid attention to the sexual health care needs of her client. She built a bridge for the client who could safely choose whether and how to respond to her enquiry. In this case the response was unexpected and complicated the nurse–patient relationship. We might consider this story as an example of the following:

◆ good practice
◆ a missed opportunity in identifying and caring for painful feelings
◆ an unexpected opportunity for care that could arise in any professional practice

◆ an opportunity for improving skills given by reflective practice and continuing training.

Case study 2.5

A woman attended for a cervical smear test. It was an everyday event for the experienced nurse, who was proud of her skills in undertaking this task competently and with as little discomfort as possible. All went well. She asked the woman, as she often did on such occasions, if all was well with love-making for her. 'It is a long time since we made love,' she said. 'My husband has cancer and had major surgery to his face and jaw; he is so disfigured that I can hardly recognise him.' The nurse indicated her concern for them both. 'He has been so ill,' the woman continued, describing her care of him. 'He said the other day, "I can't even kiss you properly."'

The nurse now found herself in a difficulty. She had been consumed by deep sympathy for the woman; now, to her discomfort, the idea of the kiss from this desperately disfigured man caught her unawares and she felt distaste and was extremely uncomfortable. Feeling guilty about her response, she finished the consultation.

The nurse reflected upon her encounter with the patient. She was troubled by what occurred and wished that she had been able to feel satisfied with her handling of the feelings she experienced. She told the story in a psychosexual training seminar she attended regularly. During discussion, the group members came to understand that these uncomfortable feelings did not belong to the nurse alone. They were probably also an accurate reflection of those experienced by the 'healthy' woman she had seen. If the nurse had felt such unease, how did the woman feel? With whom might she discuss the alienation she was experiencing from her disfigured and loved husband? Likewise, if the nurse, who did not know the man, felt guilty at her response, how might his wife be feeling and who would listen to her?

We note how the nurse's good practice of enquiring about love-making led to an unexpected outcome. She received a reply full of human suffering about the woman and her partner. The nurse was filled with compassion but also was left feeling very uncomfortable. She did, however, have the support and supervision of a seminar group, where she might discuss and understand her practice and her feelings.

Some observations on the work with feelings

We now have the opportunity to reflect upon the feelings experienced by the nurse. First, consider the powerful sense of compassion she felt. She used

> **Reflection point 2.4**
>
> You might like to use this story in discussion with colleagues or to make some reflective notes for yourself.
>
> ◆ Remember that this was an experienced nurse; she was nevertheless caught out by the complexity of the feelings.
> ◆ Do you find yourself being judgemental – if so, of whom?
> ◆ How would you have liked to respond to this patient?
> ◆ How might this nurse's unease have been understood by her and made of use at the time for the woman in her distress?
> ◆ Does this story remind you of anything from your own practice?
> ◆ How might you learn something from this story of a tragedy in a marriage, that enables you to work with the psychosexual feelings of 'healthy' people you meet in practice?

compassion to remain close to the woman whilst she spoke of the pain and distress of her husband's illness and her tiredness and stress at caring for him. The nurse was able to understand and knew she had no need to reassure the woman. She remained alongside her and showed by her professional demeanour that she understood her distress and its appropriateness to the occasion. However, the nurse began to feel uncomfortable when the woman described her husband's shattered face and his expressed wish to kiss his wife. She experienced surprising feelings of disgust and felt guilty about that. She found these unwanted feelings too difficult to deal with and brought the consultation to a close.

It is interesting to consider that the difference was that some feelings were more acceptable to this health care worker than others. That is, compassion, understanding and patience not only felt comfortable, but were shown and shared in the clinical encounter, whereas disgust and guilt proved too difficult. No longer could they be seen as shared feelings, but the nurse took them to herself, judged them there and wanted to get rid of them. The consultation closed. (See also Chapter 4, A hierarchy of feelings.)

Some practitioners might see recognition of discomfort with feelings as an opportunity to reopen the bridge for the patient, which is about to be closed by the ending of the consultation. The practitioner may consider that the uncomfortable feelings throw light upon their relationship with the client and upon her feelings too. They may consider how to make an offer, which is not a list of questions but gives opportunity for the woman to speak about what troubles her.

The practitioner and patient might decide to meet again to discuss how she is managing as time goes along.

Reflection point 2.5

◆ Can you make a list of which feelings you find most comfortable and easiest to tolerate in your work with people?

◆ Which feelings do you find most difficult?

◆ When this happens, have you ever stopped to consider where the feelings might have originated?

◆ How could you discover whether they came from the patient or yourself?

◆ How might you use your understanding to develop the way you respond?

You might like to list the ways that you could test the origins of the feelings you experience when working with people in your practice, i.e. do they originate in you or the patient?

Psychosexual awareness

Building bridges for patients and others to cross in safety

To summarise the work of this chapter, perhaps it is in the development of professional confidence that we may discover the key to psychosexual awareness:

◆ the confidence to be available to respond with closeness to another
◆ the confidence to emerge from behind the defence of knowledge with the humility to listen
◆ the confidence to take the risk of listening without the certainty of answers.

Awareness does not demand that we demonstrate what we know. Awareness is not about giving advice drawn from our fund of experience, or about knowing better than the patient; it is more. Awareness is offering the professional self to work alongside the patient in trying to understand. The wholeness of recovery and health includes the person's feelings about themselves, their sexuality and their place in society. As we develop the confidence to work with feelings that will match the confidence we feel with physical care, we can then begin to see that our role in sexual health care is of extreme importance.

Nichols (1993) demonstrates that in a renal unit, recovery is aided by staff who take responsibility for the psychological health of severely ill patients. He gives examples of success and failure when this work is addressed and when it is neglected.

The outcome of medical treatments for hypertension and diabetes are improved when the practitioner manages to understand what is important to the patient – that is, when there is empathic closeness (Kaplan et al). Patients with coronary artery disease showed greater reduction in psychological distress, systolic blood pressure, heart rate and cholesterol level when they received psychosocial intervention (Linden et al 1996). The professional use of 'self' in psychosexual care has still to be researched.

The metaphor of building bridges in care relationships

It is suggested in this chapter and others that one of the tasks of the health care professional is to build bridges that patients may cross in safety to share their feelings about what is happening to them. The strongest bridges are those where not only the patient but also the worker reaches out, each aware of the unexpressed need of the patient. Unfortunately the patient is sometimes left alone, desperately stretching towards the understanding and help that they need. On these occasions the worker may have been too busy to understand or fully appreciate a patient's cautiously expressed desire for help. At other times it may be the worker who, recognising the need of the patient to talk about the psychological pain, distress or embarrassment being experienced, bravely reaches across the void to make an offer of help. Sometimes the patient may not be ready to accept this offer. The choice is the patient's.

Franz Kafka (1992) wrote a short story in which he had the fantasy of himself as a bridge across a chasm. Preoccupied with waiting to be crossed, his terror rose. Because of that terror, when someone came to cross, he turned to view them and hurtled down. Beware the anxiety that destroys the bridge before it has been crossed!

A bridge once built does not automatically make the subsequent work easy. However, the resulting relationship can provide a structure to support future work.

Reflection point 2.6

Take some time to review the notes you have made whilst reading this chapter. Do you think that you have been relating the reading to your own clinical responsibilities? If so, what effect will your thinking have upon your practice? Do you have teaching responsibilities? How will they be affected by your thinking?

◆ What has interested you about this chapter?

◆ Have you found anything difficult?

◆ What effect upon your practice will your reading and reflections have?

◆ Was anything missing that you had hoped to read?

BIBLIOGRAPHY

You may find it useful in thinking about caring for sexuality in health to consider both the body/mind approach and the possible effects of childbirth upon the sexual health of a couple.

Skrine R 1997 Blocks and freedoms in sexual life. Radcliffe, Oxford
In Chapter 1, A Psychosexual Body/Mind Approach, the work of listening, advice and reassurance is addressed, and in Chapter 8, Sex and Childbirth, issues about feelings relevant to many practitioners in this work are raised.

Andrews G 1997 Women's sexual health. Baillière Tindall, London
In Chapter 6, Sexuality during Pregnancy, Gillian Aston has helpful information and thinking relevant to midwives, obstetric and gynaecology physiotherapists and health visitors.

Zilbergeld B 1999 The new male sexuality. Bantam, New York
Working with men about their sexuality is sometimes difficult for women practitioners. There is a consequent risk that men's difficulties may be ignored. This text is useful and helpful, giving insights into the uncertainties experienced by many men in their sexual lives.

REFERENCES

Broom B 1997 Somatic illness and the patient's other story. Free Association Books, London
Holloway R 1997 Dancing on the edge. Harper Collins, London
Kafka F 1992 The complete short stories. The Bridge. Minerva, London
Kaplan S, Greenfield S, Ware J 1989 Assessing the effects of physician–patient interactions on the outcomes of chronic disease. Medical Care 27(3) (suppl)
Linden W, Stossel C, Maurice J 1996 Psychosocial interventions for patients with coronary artery disease. A meta-analysis. Archives of Internal Medicine 156: 741–752
Nichols K 1993 (reprinted 1996) Psychological care in physical illness. Chapman & Hall, London, Ch 4, pp 58–59; Ch 5, p 113
Sadgrove J 1997 Speech therapy. Guardian (Health), 22 April
Snow J 1994 Are we doing enough? Journal of the Association of Chartered Physiotherapists in Obstetrics and Gynaecology 15: 1–2
United Kingdom Central Council for Nursing, Midwifery and Health Visiting (UKCC) 1990 Post Registration Education and Practice Project. UKCC, London
Waterhouse J, Metcalfe M 1991 Attitudes towards nurses discussing sexual concerns with patients. Journal of Advanced Nursing 16: 1048–1054

3

The courage to listen

Doreen Clifford

KEY ISSUES

- ◆ Acknowledging individuality
- ◆ Getting to know and working with patients
- ◆ The requirement of personal space in mutuality of care
- ◆ Reviewing care and saying goodbye
- ◆ The complexity of caring skills
- ◆ Caring for different groups of people and recognizing their needs
- ◆ Responsibilities for management in supporting care

INTRODUCTION

The courage to listen is not just in the moment – it is affected by the relationship with a particular patient, in a particular time or place. Therefore this chapter will discuss the practitioner–patient relationship and specific patient/client groups.

One person has many selves

From Florence Nightingale's *Notes for Nurses* first published in 1859 until today, there is an acknowledged and logical prerequisite that care must begin from a commitment to meeting the needs of the individual. One way of exploring both professional and patient needs is to recognise the many different 'selves' which make up the person. These include the physical, social, sexual, intellectual, professional, spiritual and emotional selves.

Whether as worker or patient, the self within the organisation is intimately affected by that psychosocial setting. Goffman's (1961) thesis is that the most important factor in forming a patient; is the institution, not his illness.

What any individual needs at any precise moment is unique. One task of the carer is to understand and respond to this. It may be dangerous to assume knowledge from previous experience, as though we can 'know' any individual's needs in this way. Such assumptions impoverish practice. In some conventional forms of practice we are not always good at asking for the patient's perceptions of what they need. This seems to be a particular difficulty when speaking of sexual health needs, an idea that will be developed later in the chapter. Yet who knows better what needs are than the individual person?

Professor Jean McFarlane told of visiting a hospital in the 1970s when ward routines had been recently changed to allow patients more sleep in the mornings. Talking to a lady in her late 80s and enquiring about her comfort, she got the reply, 'Well, it's alright but the nurses are lazy these days'. The patient went on to explain, 'When I was in this ward 10 years ago, we were washed, beds made and eating breakfast by half past six. These days they don't even take our temperatures until half past seven' (J Mcfarlane, unpublished work, 1974).

This amusing story of misunderstanding is worth another look. For the patient, life had been hard. Her work had begun early morning and continued until late. For her, the changes in routine were perceived as evidence of lack of willingness to care. One might ponder, what were the needs of this patient? Would a simple explanation have been valuable? Who but Jean McFarlane, until that moment, had made any enquiry about her experiences and needs?

Recognising the individual self

Whether within the setting of the hospital, clinic, surgery or the community, the task of the health care professional is to aid the patient to recover the wholeness of their 'sexual self', which is likely to be affected by the institution. It is often difficult to function fully in a strange place with which one is not familiar. It is too easy to become unnecessarily humble or even uncharacteristically belligerent in the face of the unknown or frighteningly new experiences.

A useful way of testing this observation is to consider what happens in the first few hours or days on holiday in a new setting, especially when by oneself. Whether in another country, when there are the adjustments of language, or just in a new area of a well known country, we are likely to feel strange and rather lost when we first arrive. We become less than ourselves, feel at a loss and are often diffident about asking for help. When looking for a particular place our observational skills are likely to fail us.

A man told of how, on a visit to New York, he was unable to find the huge United Nations building. He stopped to ask a policeman who pointed over his shoulder. They were standing directly in front of it!

Most of us may have experienced such things happening when in a new and strange place. Embarking on the course for our chosen profession is another useful memory to explore. Connect this to the experience of someone entering your setting – a 'country' to which they are unaccustomed and where the 'language' is not familiar to them. (When we find *ourselves* as patients in a new setting, this may give us fresh insights into patient care.)

Given that a person who has become a patient finds herself in a new setting, how do the professionals respond most helpfully? How best is the person helped to feel fully adult, comfortable to be herself whilst still able to regress into that state her complaint or illness makes of her?

Imagine a worker who is in someone's home in the community. On a first visit, when unaccustomed to the family and the setting, how quickly is she able to recover her professional self and confidence? Her full self enables her to be available to the family and not find it necessary to retire and be diminished with a flattened 'persona', less than herself. This chapter will attempt to explore some of these themes.

GETTING TO KNOW PATIENTS

Saying 'hello' and building new relationships

First meetings are vital in building relationships of trust. The importance of the first meeting with a patient cannot be overemphasised. It is during the first meeting that the alliance to work together to regain sexual health or function is begun. An approach that leaves patient and worker confident of their own selfhood is the most valuable.

At first meetings information-giving is often important. However, this needs careful consideration. Sometimes the practitioner spends much of the time providing information they hope will 'reassure'; but the patient has little opportunity to express their concerns. The 'there is nothing to worry about' approach is likely to interfere with important understandings.

There is so much to do at a first meeting. Information to give, information to collect and checks on understandings by both parties. This is the formal procedure. The informal work is the 'sizing up' that occurs: 'What kind of worker, what kind of client is this'?

Recognising the wide variety of times health care workers are able to spend with patients and the differing opportunities available is interesting. Times may vary from brief encounters of a few minutes, to the other extreme of long relationships of many years duration, and all that goes between. This is not simple work. The professional needs to be able to develop the ability to 'think on her feet'. Sometimes referred to as 'reflection in action' (Schon 1987), this requires daily work and skills to be reviewed regularly and thoughtfully. Such reflections during and upon practice are a necessity if we are to maintain standards of care in responding to clients as individuals and developing confidence to do so (see Section 3, Seminar training).

The following was written by a nurse reflecting on working in a busy family planning clinic.

Case study 3.1

'Sometimes I get wrong footed with a patient by making an inappropriate jokey comment when making initial introductions. I am conscious that I need to watch this as I realise that it sometimes makes it more difficult for the patient to say what's on her mind and this has an adverse influence on the nurse–patient relationship.

I do try to think of how I appear to the patient, i.e. if I were a patient would I want to see *me* as a nurse. If I am irritated by someone, for instance if they are slow to answer questions and I realise I'm getting testy, I try to stop and explain why I am asking for this information, which usually improves the situation and they become more cooperative. There is so much to do in the first interview, particularly if it is for emergency contraception: there is the presenting history, the need to review the risk contraceptively and from a sexual infection perspective, information to give about alternative methods of emergency contraception; and future contraception to be discussed and maybe taught. In with this there may be other physical or psychosexual problems that may need addressing. This is often an emergency patient and there will be four or five more women waiting to be seen.

What can be seen from this piece is the nurse's consciousness that how she approaches a patient can make all the difference to the outcome for them both. She sees that initial mistakes can be rectified if the needs of the patient are borne in mind even in a pressured situation, e.g. stopping to explain when she finds herself irritated by a patient's seeming slowness (see also Chapter 4, Keeping a reflective diary).

Reflection point 3.1

Questions to ask oneself and reflect upon after the first meeting:

◆ Does the new patient have a view of my 'professional self' that leaves them with confidence about their stay in this institution or our work together in the clinic or community?

◆ Do I have a picture of this person as a functioning adult in their own life, no matter how they look or how ill or troubled they are at this moment? If not, am I confident of making space to discover this whilst offering care during the coming time together?

◆ Is there anything to be learned from the feelings that I already have about this person that might help me understand them better? Are the feelings comfortable or am I left somewhat uneasy? What can I learn from this to help in my clinical work?

Sensitivity to gay and lesbian people

It is often during longer relationships with patients that opportunities occur to recognise both gay and lesbian people (see Chapter 10). Hospitalisation and long-term illness disrupt sexual feelings, relationships and responses for everyone. Opportunities to talk about the feelings involved are important.

Case study 3.2

Alice, who was caring for her dying partner, spoke of the relief she felt when together they told one member of the hospice staff of their lesbian relationship. They wanted other staff to know and so gave their permission for the practitioner to inform her colleagues. Then like other couples they could be supported by the staff, privacy was ensured and Alice shared in the intimate care of her loved one.

Further reading to stimulate your thinking about the health care needs of gay and lesbian people is listed in the annotated bibliography at the end of the chapter.

Working together and attempting to hear

At times of psychosexual transition an individual may require help in re-assessing and understanding changes in her sexual self. It is then that the skills of listening for requests for help are needed.

Reflection point 3.2

◆ What is your view of the sexual feelings and needs of gay and lesbian people in hospitals and hospices where you work?

◆ Why do you think there seems to be a reluctance to reveal sexual orientation?

◆ Do you work in the community? How do you attempt to meet the needs of the gay and lesbian people you meet in your practice?

◆ Do you give due attention to homosexual people of either sex in your care? Have you considered learning to improve your professional skills by discussing the perceptions of a gay patient or client?

◆ Do you always identify patients as 'straight' or do you make it part of your assessment to enable people to express their sexual identity? What ideas do you have about the need for confidentiality?

◆ When seeking next-of-kin, how would you address this issue with a person you are admitting to hospital? What about the 'friend' accompanying?

◆ Did you know that many gay and lesbian people actively fear discrimination in hospital treatment?

Ordinary events occurring in health such as the menarche, puberty, the beginning of sexual relationships, childbirth, parenting, changes of sexual partner, the menopause and growing older all require recognition as occasions likely to trigger times of disruption. There is a place here for the health care worker to support the person through the transition so that their healthy sexual functioning is soon resumed. Many health visitors have experience of this. Later difficulties may be forestalled by such intervention, thus saving time and energy (see Reflection points 3.6 and 3.7 following Robert's story on pp 56–57).

The area many health care workers find challenging is that of recognising and taking responsibility for working with the individual's sexual self, i.e. taking care of that part of the person's feelings likely to have been disrupted by ill health, including feelings about their sexual relationships. Disruptions to the sexual self may occur during any illness, hospital admission or treatment. Recognising that feelings are disrupted on these occasions is the first step towards understanding the need to listen. The worker is not required to know the answers. Rather, the task is to provide a space in which the patient may share aloud with the worker troubling concerns and anxieties.

Building bridges for worker and patient to meet

In the previous chapters there are several references to 'bridge building' for patients. This useful metaphor was developed by a group of nurses who met regularly in a psychosexual training seminar. It gradually became clear to members that the opportunity to communicate and understand seemed to flower when the link between nurse and patient was efficient and trustworthy. Thus developed the shorthand phrase 'bridge building' to describe the mutual and agreed sharing that followed. Each reached out towards the other and met in safety to work together on the task of understanding.

Part of the sensitivity to respond to the patient's tentative reaching out to speak on sensitive issues depends upon the worker–client relationship. This is a complex transaction. Berne (1968) writes of the personality having, as it were, three 'parts' – parent, adult and child – a concept that can clarify some difficult interactions in daily practice (Fig. 3.1).

Viewed in this way many complexities and misunderstandings in communications between practitioner and client become clearer. For example, when relationships develop as if between a 'parental' worker and a 'child-like' patient (Fig. 3.2), who is diminished by such a relationship? When communication is between two adults, the complexity is eased and mutuality in the task can be agreed (Fig. 3.3).

Part of sensitivity in responding to the patient's tentative reaching out to speak on intimate issues depends upon space in the worker–client relationship. The concept of space between the attentive listening worker and the patient offers both the opportunity to think about their feelings. Casement (1990) writes of how the mental and emotional space between people can be eroded by the claims that each makes upon the other, and points out the therapeutic potential of space. Penman (1998), discussing the care of patients with sexual anxieties, shows that when there exists a

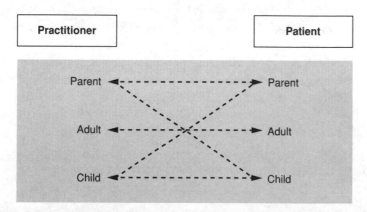

Fig. 3.1 The possibility of complex interactions

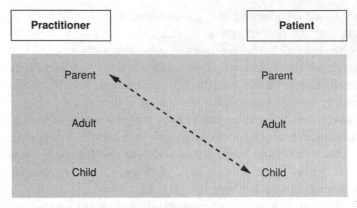

Fig. 3.2 Diminished 'child-like' patient and 'parental' worker

therapeutic space between an 'unknowing' worker and client, the opportunity is offered for the client to begin to discover the connection between their emotions and bodily (sexual) symptoms. That is, when the worker can tolerate not knowing the answers, a space is available for the patient. In this way there is opportunity for the patient to think and put together ideas and understandings about their feelings of psychosexual disruption (Fig. 3.4).

Value lies in the attempt to maintain a co-equal therapeutic working relationship, where understandings that arise are a mutual discovery. We can discover the benefit for the patient of having space for consideration of their own feelings and understandings in several examples in this Section.

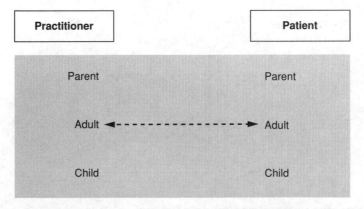

Fig. 3.3 Mutuality is working together to understand

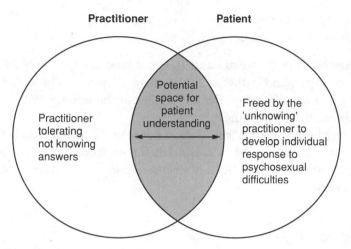

Practitioner   **Patient**

Potential space for patient understanding

Practitioner tolerating not knowing answers

Freed by the 'unknowing' practitioner to develop individual response to psychosexual difficulties

Fig. 3.4 Space for the patient

Testing out trust with each other

An imagined, unspoken conversation is a suggestion of the queries that occupy patient and worker when testing out trustworthiness. Each thought and idea occupies but a nanosecond and does not interrupt the conversation.

The *patient's* questions are a kind of testing of the relationship when considering putting their vulnerable self on offer:

◆ Is it safe?
◆ Is it permissible to talk about intimate feelings?
◆ Will this worker listen and understand?
◆ Will it help the difficulty I am in?

The *worker's* response is also likely to be tentative:

◆ Do I want to listen?
◆ Do I have time?
◆ Do I have the courage to listen?
◆ Have I the necessary skills – will I be expected to know the answers?

Something similar happens when the *worker* proffers the bridge framework:

◆ Will this offer be understood?
◆ Will this person be offended?
◆ Will I understand the response?

The *patient* must make decisions, for example:

◆ Am I understanding this question aright?
◆ Is it an offer to talk about intimate feelings?

◆ Am I ready to do this yet?
◆ Is this the worker I would have chosen?

Whenever the professional makes the offer, however appropriate it may be, the choice to respond is always for the client to make. As in Kafka's (1992) short story about the bridge, the anxiety lies in the waiting. Will the bridge be strong enough to hold the burden?

A strong bridge requires cooperation between the bridge builders. When the patient reaches out, the worker needs the professional skills to respond. To the patient belongs the choice of whether or not to use the offer of a meeting on a bridge.

Saying goodbye

'Every time we say goodbye, I cry a little. Every time we say goodbye I die a little', says the song.

How do you say farewell to relatives and friends who leave your home? Most of us do it by seeing them to their transport and waving them off and wishing them a safe journey. Should a stay in a hospital be so very different and shouldn't we show care in a similar way?

Saying goodbye is as important as saying hello in clinical care. Why is it then that so little respect is given to this important clinical event in the experience of many? 'There is no time for such frills these days,' some might say. Some workers still say goodbye with a small ceremony, for example, carrying a patient's bag and escorting them to the door of the unit. Such an event may confirm the importance of the relationship in clinical care. In the community, some practitioners consider it an integral part of their professionalism to shake hands in farewell when completing a period of care. Some maternity units make it their norm for baby and parents to be accompanied to waiting transport by a member of staff and waved off.

Indeed, clinical care is time-consuming from beginning to end, as we have been observing in this chapter. As we have also seen, quality of care rests upon the recognition of and response to the individual. So perhaps it is the 'farewell ceremony' of going over and reliving the patient's experience of their stay that is the truly important clinical event. As one man said in tribute to his practitioner when leaving the unit where he had made a recovery from a severe HIV illness, 'Maybe I can have a life.'

One of the reasons for the failure to recognize the importance of goodbyes seems to lie in the lack of respect that some workers have for their own individuality and worth. Do you say goodbye to patients when going off duty, going away for days off, moving to a different ward? Do you tell a patient that you will not be there when you have been giving them special care and are going to be away? Why is that?

It may be that the practitioner's own clinical worth is not properly valued. When this happens, is it any surprise that other professionals find it difficult to value the health care worker?

In coming to the end of a particular period of treatment or time in hospital, the value of 'review' cannot be over emphasized. It is important to round off an experience as a patient by reviewing that time with a health care professional. The memory of the experience and the feelings involved need recognition. It is also an opportunity to express gratitude and grumbles about treatment and the recognition of the current health situation with hopes and fears for the future.

The development and use of this way of reviewing an experience to bring it to completion, is an important therapeutic device in every area of health care. This is also an opportunity to reflect upon the insights that emerge about one's own practice.

The therapeutic nature of review

The therapeutic nature of reflection upon the events and feelings of a patient's experience is not uniquely the patient's. It is also an opportunity for the practitioner to share in the reflective process so that it becomes a dialogue and an opportunity to learn something about one's own practice (see Chapter 4, The patient as coach). Reflection could confirm or suggest appropriate changes to current skills.

There may be changes to recommend in the institution. During your review with this patient, was anything said that you consider would contribute to the well-being of the organisation as a whole? The Patient's Charter invites complaints, compliments or suggestions about the service received. Should the patient be encouraged to write to report their experience? Perhaps these suggestions would be better dealt with by information to immediate colleagues and staff with management responsibilities. Shepherd (1994) did some interesting research on patients' views following their discharge. She helped inpatients to express their views by telling them what people who were discharged sometimes said.

Saying goodbye can be viewed as an opportunity for patients, their partners or families, to consider the treatment process recently experienced. It provides practitioners with the opportunity to have a fresh view of their clinical practice and can provide insights into management practices from the point of view of the user of the service, the patient. People with power in the institution can be kept informed of successes and failures in their domain when patients write to give accounts of their experiences.

DIFFERENT OPPORTUNITIES IN CLINICAL ENCOUNTERS

Opportunities to offer sexual health care to patients happen in a number of settings. All clinical places where professional health care workers and clients meet are an opportunity to listen for clues to people seeking recognition of their wish to discuss their feelings in some way.

Some physical care giving is brief, in A & E for example. Some is intense, e.g. during acute and severe illness and following accidents. There are other worker–client relationships, during longer term care, e.g. people with disabilities, patients in urology units, during cancer care, or in orthopaedic departments. And then there are occasional and brief encounters.

Brief encounters

Well men and well women clinics are places where client and workers meet briefly, with long intervals between. The client attends clinic or surgery once every few years for weight and blood pressure checks. There are real opportunities here to ask about sexual health issues. Quite simple questions like 'is making love going well for you', or 'is there anything you would like to discuss about your love-making whilst you are here?' may be asked. Such words may be all someone needs to talk over feelings with someone who will try to understand. Maybe you already use a phrase to which a client could respond easily. Sometimes it is enough to offer conversational 'space' in which the client may indicate their wish to talk.

Genitourinary and gynaecological outpatient clinics are also occasions when many men and women might welcome the opportunity to spend a few moments discussing particular sexual worries.

Case study 3.3

Mrs Johnson attended the clinic complaining of bladder pain. She said it was so severe that it interfered with everything she did. Her baby girl, who accompanied her, was a charming 6-month-old. The nurse asked about her. Mrs Johnson said the pain dated back to her birth.

Following full examination nothing abnormal was discovered. Things seemed at a standstill until the nurse thought to ask whether the phrase 'interferes with everything I do' included love-making too. Mrs Johnson started weeping and said that since the baby's birth she could not make love. The birth had been very painful and she did not want to make love any more because of the pain. She was then seen by the doctor who referred her for psychosexual counselling.

Perhaps you do not feel sufficiently experienced to respond. It may be that you still feel that you do not yet have the confidence to ask and still require to give that perfect response.

This is an example of a clinical nurse specialist in continence care, with no psychosexual training, whose response enabled a woman to receive help.

Mrs Johnson's story shows a good example of the nurse's listening skills even though the nurse had not had the confidence to do this before. She has since joined a psychosexual training seminar and feels that in similar circumstances she herself would now spend time with a patient like Mrs Johnson before deciding whether further referral was necessary.

Longer working relationships

Opportunities to listen carefully and indeed to make helpful enquiries may more easily occur when there has been time to build trust during longer working relationships. Cancer care, for example, gives opportunities to get to know patients well. There is opportunity to recognise an appropriate time to open a discussion on how the illness has affected feelings or produced problems in loving (Cort, 1998).

Case study 3.4

One worker told of opening a discussion about psychosexual issues with a 17-year-old woman by quite simply asking whether she had a boyfriend. What she heard in response and listened to, was the patient's pain about his unwillingness to visit her during her term of chemotherapy. She missed him a great deal but found it difficult to have opportunities to talk about him as her parents disapproved of the relationship continuing during her illness.

Reflection point 3.3

Please set aside some time to consider this story carefully. Does it remind you of anything in your own area of work that you find challenging? You could reflect upon this and make notes considering opportunities you have not yet explored for developing skills to respond to the psychosexual needs of your patients.

◆ Why might the parents of this patient have resisted the relationship with the young man?

◆ Can you see any interventions by the worker that could have helped the situation?

◆ Do you have responsibilities to care for younger people?

◆ Do you consider patient's sexual feelings and needs to be your responsibility?

◆ How do you address this in your own practice?

Many people with long-term illnesses such as asthma, heart disease, urological illnesses and degenerative diseases would welcome opportunities to discuss how their sexual lives are physically restrained by illness and how feelings about their partnership are affected.

Intermittent and longer working relationships

Some professional relationships could be described as 'long and thin', i.e. they sometimes continue for many months or even years. It is possible to meet the same people over a number of years in hospital outpatient and treatment clinics; the patients may have problems ranging from varicose ulcers to asthma care, or diabetes to a chronic chest condition. Similarly, in the community, some workers know their patients for years. GP surgeries maintain many patients, some are hardly ever seen, some frequently and some attend for regular checks and treatments.

Opportunities to recognise and respond to sexual health care needs are an important part of such professional relationships. However, given pressure of work and reluctance to voice such issues, it is all too easy to avoid this work. When knowing patients for some time it is easy to slip into taking for granted that a patient seen regularly always feels the same, always has the same needs. The unspoken pain of some people fails to be addressed and their feelings are hidden away when met by the hearty method of greeting used by some practitioners when under pressure. This seems to keep people at bay and real, mutually adult relationships can be cheerfully avoided. Do you recognise this practice?

In some circumstances it may be difficult to make a space for each individual to be herself. Time is never too short, however, to take the opportunity to ask, 'What can I do for you today?' or make some similar approach. Some practice nurses find that this gives opportunity to talk about fresh needs and any current worries. Sometimes the response we call forth is surprising, as in Mr Blake's story.

Case study 3.5

The practice nurse met with Mr Blake, whom she had known for 18 months. He was a short, rosy-faced man who attended regularly for a blood pressure check. On this occasion he asked if he could talk about something difficult. He looked away as he said, very quietly, 'I find it difficult to keep it up.' The nurse had to lean forwards to hear. She suddenly realised he was referring to his penis. Shocked and in some disarray, the nurse turned to her computer to check what drugs he was receiving. Avoiding eye contact, she referred him back to the GP for reconsideration of his drug regime.

The nurse reported this encounter in a psychosexual seminar. When she considered this meeting in the context of her earlier relationship with Mr Blake, she realised he did not usually look away when talking and she did not usually face her computer when talking to him. It was only on this occasion. Both of them were embarrassed and this inhibited her from giving care in any way other than referring him to someone else.

THE DEVELOPMENT OF SKILLS

The need for bravery

Anxiety

When beginning to venture into this work, and whilst developing confidence in the professional use of self, we tend to become driven by anxiety. Anxiety can produce a 'busy' worker and inhibit responses. Courage is the element required by the person beginning to initiate talk of sexual feelings with patients. The *Concise Oxford Dictionary* defines courage as 'the ability to disregard fear'. Fear of a variety of kinds is the most quoted reason for disregarding the sexual self of the patient. How do we understand the feelings inhibiting us? It seems likely that the trouble stems from misunderstanding.

Waterhouse & Metcalfe (1991), in their research, have shown that the majority of patients would like nurses (and, we may extrapolate, other workers) to initiate talk about sexuality with them.

Some health care workers have expressed fear that their recognition of 'sexuality' will lead them into dangerous pathways where they may be misunderstood by patients and by colleagues. They fear accusations of inappropriate behaviour. They appear afraid that if they ask about the sexual aspect of the patient's self, they will touch off responses with which they cannot deal and that psychosexual awareness will demand actions that they are unable and unwilling to undertake. It is important that we understand this response if we are to offer appropriate support and training to such workers.

Some practitioners who work in isolation have described the difficulties of coping with inappropriate sexual behaviour. Replies to a questionnaire to physiotherapists in New South Wales raised concern and issues about future training (Weerakoon & O'Sullivan 1998).

Media influences

In our society, press, television and the media generally, present sexuality as something always active, usually about intercourse of several kinds. They describe boundless sexual appetites, extraordinary genital athleticism, gold medal and multiple orgasms. Zilbergeld (1999, Ch 2) refers to this as 'the fantasy model of sex'. It often seems that the tentative first kiss, holding hands, shyness, sharing and cuddling, i.e. the ordinary events of loving, are too insignificant to merit attention.

In light of this bombardment of what 'fantasy' sexuality is, it is not easy to keep an awareness of the minor, everyday acts of sexuality that can be observed in the course of clinical practice. For example, a couple talking softly together at the bedside over the head of their new baby, two men holding hands whilst a chemotherapy infusion runs through into an arm, a partner who wishes to wash and toilet their dying 'other', may all be demonstrating sexual love. Recognising the disturbance of feeling at times such as these is the business of the professional worker. This is the ordinary, rather than extra-ordinary, sexuality of daily life.

We might question just how this understanding is best achieved. It is in a variety of ways that each worker must discover for herself and depends upon the practitioner–patient relationship, the type of work and the place in which it happens.

The work of understanding

The concept of 'understanding' too easily becomes confused by the desire to know, the need to find out. Perhaps this once again links with our training. This brings us to the use of questions. The problem with questions is that they only get answers. That is, the question itself can be a trap, it may be the wrong thing to ask to get the knowledge one is seeking. Professionals become so used to collecting clinical information by means of question and answer that the method is in danger of moving into every clinical encounter. The art of listening to understand is a skill many workers use extensively without necessarily recognising either that they have it or how skilful it is (see Section 3 for accounts of this work developed through seminar training).

Patients also ask questions and once one has grown used to the idea that 'something tends to lie behind a question', the more interesting the questions can become. A question as simple as 'Why do I need an X-ray?' may mean 'I only had one last week', or it may indicate a worry about tuberculosis from which this person's father died, or be as complex as fear of serious illness or worries about radiation. It is usually worth enquiring, 'Why do you ask?' as well as giving an answer.

Questioning

Some hospitals use computers for patients to fill in details of themselves. Sometimes this is done by practitioners. No doubt this provides an efficient and time-saving way of data collection but there is a danger of cutting down the time spent in clinical interaction. Importantly, one might ask, 'Is the time saved used with the patient? Is it spent on learning more from the patient about the effect of illness upon their life?' The complexities of disease and ill health are more likely to become clear in the interpersonal interactions of conversation. The aim of sexual health care is to develop understanding of the distress, trouble and anxiety, together with the patient.

Non-verbal communications

Touch

Touch in all its forms makes its mark on our health from birth, and the need for human contact is one of the fundamental desires shaping human behaviour. Many women from the Indian sub-continent, for example, as a matter of course massage their babies when they are restless or crying, to help them relax and sleep. In other cultures, rocking, singing lullabies and cuddling are used in comforting babies. Winnicott (1969) writes of 'the close connection that there is between the physiotherapy of men and women of any age and the early care that a mother is able to give her baby.'

Practitioners' use of touch is often highly skilled and has been described as a form of embodied knowledge (Savage 1995). When this is observed and discussed by practitioners the unconscious can be made conscious, helping in skill development.

Recognition of the individuality of the patient is demonstrated by the cues in communication given by where one sits, e.g. alongside the patient or on the bed or by holding a hand or touching a knee. Patients often respond to clues in non-verbal communication when, for example, a practitioner makes eye contact in a way that says, 'I am here to listen to you'. It is in such professionalising of touch, that health care workers have gone on to develop for themselves in professional encounters, that skills come to be embodied.

Two different kinds of touching An important part of the skills of a health care worker lies in the training to touch to bring comfort and cleanliness, and relief from pain and discomfort, but many other professionals fail to see the value of this work. This is why it is important that health care workers recognise and integrate into their sense of professionalism such tasks as bathing, toiletting and the simple use of touch, e.g. holding someone's hand when speaking to them directly. We need to draw the attention of management colleagues to these skills as of high importance in the health care professions. Embodied knowledge is as important as skilful surgery.

The professional health care worker has the privilege of touching another person as a part of the working task. Savage (1995) describes two categories of 'everyday' touch in professional care: *expressive touch* (sometimes called caring or comforting touch) and *instrumental touch* (alternatively referred to as task-orientated or procedural touch).

Case study 3.6

Mrs Simpson's hand had been amputated and she was recovering in hospital. This was a distressing time for her and she spent a lot of time weeping. The consultant surgeon who had operated on her did a ward round, inspected the wound and taught the group with him about the procedure he had used. He told Mrs Simpson how well she was doing and how pleased he was with the operation.

Mrs Simpson was devastated, she felt 'alone and like a window mannequin'. Quite suddenly, the ward sister left the entourage and came back to see her. She sat on the bed, held her other hand and said, 'I am so sorry that you had to lose your hand.' She went on to explain some of the reasons for the necessity of the procedure. The humanity of the touch was the turning point of Mrs Simpson's recovery.

The skill of touching another person in a professional way may lead to surprising confidences. Sometimes the response is of relief to have found someone with whom they can share the feeling that, e.g. 'the loving is not quite right'. Many community midwives, for example, hear details of a woman's intimate life following delivery, and requests for help are sometimes received on such occasions. Sometimes, of course, we can stop someone speaking, by a touch on an arm, for instance, or offering tissues to a weeping person.

The trust of the ill or disabled patient rests in the professional touch for ease of distress, even when a painfully infected wound needs cleaning. This trust is part of the reward we have for our professional skills. Achieving such confidence is one of the ways of getting in touch with some of the many 'selves' of our patients.

It is whilst attending with touch to a patient that the opportunity to disclose painful feelings and worries of a sexual nature may arise, including disturbances to sexual feelings and relationships. At such times the practitioner needs to be particularly alert to the 'reaching out' that may emerge, disguised, in the conversation. Sometimes the space is occupied by silence that encourages someone to attempt to talk over their difficulties. The test is whether the worker will take flight.

Because of basic insecurities about sex and our sensitivity to anything sexual it is sometimes difficult to have the courage to clarify with the patient how they would like us to respond. Remember that your insecurities, shyness and sensitivities are also a reflection of the patient's feelings. Such uncomfortable feelings are a part of common humanity, but it is the task of the professional worker to respond.

Troubled memories Sacks (1986) writes of his experience of the body actually having memory that maintains function. Touch triggers memories in many of us and for some this may prove difficult. Kitzinger (1990) quotes this story:

'We were catheterising an old, blind woman, she must have been about 90. It took four nurses to carry out the procedure – three of us were needed to hold her down. And all this old woman was saying was, 'Please don't do it daddy, please don't do it daddy.' We all went silent. It was never discussed, nobody dared mention it.'

The nurse who described this incident to me was very distressed that there was no support either for the woman or for the staff. We do not know what the woman herself thought. However, from my interviews with 39 survivors of childhood sexual abuse (women between the ages of 16 and 59) it is clear that medical procedures can often bring back overwhelming memories of sexual violence.

Kitzinger suggests that professionals need to be alert to patients who 'become uncooperative' and disrupt busy routines when internal examinations are needed. Such fears of minor procedures can seem irrational. Staff may feel at a loss as to how to respond to a woman's distress, thereby feeling undermined in their professional role. Kitzinger suggests that many such patients may be associating the examination with previous abuse and sexual violence. She goes on to say that treatment from caring and sensitive practitioners can enable the patient to develop a more nurturing relationship with their own body. Indeed, Kitzinger believes that health workers have a vital role in ensuring that treatment counteracts, rather than reinforces, the effects of sexual violence.

Reflection point 3.4

◆ Why was the extremely disturbing and painful effect of the woman's words so difficult for the nurses involved to discuss?

◆ Do you think it might be the 'unspeakable' nature of the underlying history that made it more difficult to talk over as a clinical difficulty?

◆ Have you ever had a clinical event that left you feeling so troubled that you have been unable to talk about it with colleagues?

◆ Could you use this printed story to raise the issue with colleagues in discussion, to try to share your own event with them? Perhaps others may have similar painful professional secrets.

◆ If you cannot do this at present, write your story for yourself to see whether you might understand your own feelings better at the time and since. Maybe this could also enable you to understand the patient's needs a little better and clarify your thinking for the future.

The professional use of touch Touch can also enrich professional closeness when caring for patients. Many professionals believe that touching and handling the bodies of ill people is itself part of the healing process. Physiotherapists are fully at ease with this skill. The challenge is to respond to the help being sought for troubled feelings. It was during an intimate examination involving touching, that the following distressing story emerged and was responded to.

Case study 3.7

A woman came to a clinic for help because she had been having painful and reluctant intercourse with her husband since their baby's birth some 3 years before. She felt something was wrong with her. Whilst examining her vagina, the nurse asked about the birth of the baby. The woman described her difficult labour which ended in a forceps delivery. She said that everyone, including herself and her husband, were anxious about the outcome.
The unborn baby was showing signs of distress. Because of this, she had numerous vaginal examinations. 'They may have all been doctors,' she said, 'I did not know, no one introduced themselves. Some were in white coats, some in shirt sleeves, one could have been the porter for all I knew.'
   She felt humiliated that her vagina had become public property and was still angry and upset with the way she was handled. Furthermore she still did not feel her vagina belonged to her yet and was unsure whether she wished it to.

Note that it was the professional touch to her vagina during the present examination which freed the woman to discuss the events that had so traumatised her sexual relationship. It was this discussion that alerted the nurse to the woman's need for psychosexual care. Delivery distress is a not uncommon complication of childbirth (Guardian 1996).

One might ask whether the woman and her husband had spent time with a midwife or doctor following this traumatic occasion. Maybe a professional person *had* listened to her story soon after the delivery, but she had no memory of this happening and had felt abandoned by the staff.

It can be difficult giving quality listening to someone who is expressing criticism of colleagues. In the face of the anxiety, even panic, in the delivery room to get the baby born alive, criticism can appear ungrateful. Yet, this woman was traumatised by what amounted to her depersonalisation during the event (see Chapter 10).

What implications are there in this story for practice? If you are a clinical team manager, a charge nurse or head of department, what regular opportunities do you arrange for your workers to talk over their professional feelings together?

Reflection point 3.5

You might like to reflect upon this patient's story and the implications for your own practice. These questions may be used in discussion with your clinical team.

◆ What has been your experience of being told something painful when touching a patient in the course of treatment?

◆ Do you offer opportunities for the patient to reflect on their experiences following illness, childbirth or surgery in your own clinical practice?

◆ When someone has recovered from serious illness or surgery, do you make opportunity to listen to what it felt like for them? How did they experience care? Supposing they are critical, how do you handle that?

◆ What opportunities are given in your professional practice to make sure every patient has the opportunity to talk over the events of birth and labour with a qualified practitioner?

◆ Is any report given to your professional team about patients' observations on the care they received?

◆ Are couples ever given the opportunity to review their experiences together with a member of staff in your practice?

◆ What is it like to listen to criticism of colleagues?

◆ What is it like to listen to praise of colleagues?

◆ What is it like to experience shame about the work of fellow professionals and how might this be of value in practice?

◆ Is the criticism or the praise of colleagues more difficult to share with the staff group – why?

THE NEEDS OF PARTICULAR GROUPS

Children

We were once all children and know that children's perceptions of events are not always those of an adult. Chapter 7 of this book offers insights into how childhood perceptions and understandings may be carried into adult life to help or hinder.

Robert's story

The following case study is an example of someone seeking covert help with a severe psychosexual problem which is ruining his life – his inability to maintain a loving sexual relationship. Behind this and many other severe and sad psychosexual problems that are presented to health care professionals, lie years of missed opportunities for help, such as adequate explanations, help by discussion and exploration of feeling, all of which ordinary professional practice could have dealt with. Such help would have saved a great deal of suffering not just for Robert but for his mother and his previous partners.

Case study 3.8

The setting is a well man clinic. The practitioner taking the history of a client in his early 30s made routine enquiry into his sexual health. The man, Robert, rather dismissively, said all was well. He'd had a number of heterosexual liaisons in the past, including one with a child. Now he had met someone with whom he would like to settle down and build a life together. The problem was, he never seemed able to maintain a commitment to a woman; after a while he had found himself drifting away, unable to maintain feelings or commitment. In fact, he said, this was probably the real reason he was there this evening.

The nurse, an experienced man, felt helpless at the carefully controlled distress shown in Robert's demeanour. He respected the feelings as Robert's, saying just how helpless Robert seemed to feel at his distressing failure to make a lasting relationship. Robert responded angrily and said that he blamed his mother. He told the nurse this story:

As a small boy, he had an operation for undescended testicles. This had not gone well and he had to be readmitted to hospital for a second operation. He said his mother had not explained or talked to him about the operation, and he had found the whole business terrifying. He had been very frightened by the hospital, the operation and the stitches. He had not understood what was happening or what it was about and had never been able to ask. When, at about 14, Robert had brought a girl home to tea, he had overheard his mother tell her that, because of an operation, he could never father a child. He was very embarrassed then and blamed that occasion for his continuing failures.

Robert was referred for psychosexual counselling. Whatever the outcome of this, and however significant the story proved to be, many questions are raised for health care workers of all disciplines.

It is interesting to examine how the nurse, who received supervision in a Balint psychosexual nursing seminar, enabled Robert to tell his story and listened so carefully. He was surprised by the intensity of the story, but thought on his feet. By recognising his own feelings of helplessness he was able to understand the intensity of Robert's similar feelings.

Reflection point 3.6

You might like to consider for yourself and/or discuss with colleagues, which professional health workers you consider could help a child coming for such surgery today with his parents.

Make a list and compare it with the following suggestions:

◆ The Health Visitor

◆ The School Nurse

◆ The Practice Nurse

◆ Staff in the Paediatric Department.

Do you consider that psychosexual awareness in the practice of the above professionals could limit similar damage to that experienced by Robert?

How do you consider each professional could best go about approaching the subject with today's 'Robert' and his parent?

Do you blame Robert's mother for his trouble? What help would you expect a parent in a similar situation would receive today?

Reflection point 3.7

In the light of Robert's story, what advice would you give to a worker admitting a child to hospital for:

◆ General surgery

◆ Surgery related to the genitals.

What pre-admission advice would you recommend and what follow-up or debriefing would you advise for the child and his parent?

Deborah Moggach (1995) published a charming short story, 'Changing Babies', which illustrates the perceptions of a small boy in distress and how this is complicated by his misunderstanding of a simple phrase. How could understanding the likelihood of different perceptions in a child inform your practice? Do you have any recent examples from your own practice with a child and a parent, which could inform the theoretical standpoints of this book?

Sexual care of the older person

In the *Guardian* newspaper there is a weekly column 'Private Lives', which deals with a problem sent in by a reader. The problem appears one week and is repeated the second week with replies from other readers. On 18 January 1999, the problem was from an older couple aged 70 and 72 who felt criticised by their family following revelations of their active and happy sexual life together. One of the respondents was Dr Sally Greengross, Director General, Age Concern, England. She wrote:

Simone de Beauvoir said, 'Old people have the same desires, the same feelings, the same requirements as the young, but the world responds with disgust.' We always see in TV, films and advertising that sex is only for the young and unwrinkled ...Sexuality is a normal part of our make-up as complex human beings and can enrich our lives and help us at any age to experience new levels of intimacy and personal fulfilment. Many couples enjoy sex more as they get older. You should be free to decide for yourselves what you need and what is right for you personally.

People with disabilities

There is an increasing recognition of the needs of people with a variety of severely disabling conditions and their requirements for recognition and help with practical sexual problems.

For further reading it is salutary to read the research into disabled women's sexuality reported by Gillespie-Sells et al (1998). The authors tell the stories of many disabled women. All the stories help to 'dispel the myth that disabled women are asexual and have no interest in forging sexual and personal relationships'.[1]

Bodily changes

Stoma care and sexuality

A recent paper highlights the need for practitioners to recognise and grow skills in responding to the psychosexual needs of people with stomas. Huish et al (1998) contend that stomas have a significant physical, emotional and psychological effect on bodily functions. They report that almost a quarter of people who have stoma operations experience serious problems with anxiety and depression at some point during the year of their stoma operation. They say that, when discussing sexuality with stoma patients, 'The intent is not to find and diagnose a problem to cure, but the focus should be on issues that are important to the patient.'

MANAGEMENT RESPONSIBILITIES FOR ENSURING CONTINUING TRAINING

Whatever political and economic forces are at work at any given time, health care workers function best with the support of continuing training. It is when people feel professionally at ease they can take responsibility for the standards

---

[1] Useful contact: SPOD, 286 Camden Road, Holloway, London N7 OBJ, UK, Tel: 0207 607 8851.

set in the organisations where they are employed. It requires confidence to bring to the attention of managers the fact that changes are required because current structures are failing to meet patients' needs.

Reflection point 3.8

After reading the above examples, make some notes for yourself on the different kinds of sexuality described in the pieces. With which are you most comfortable and why?

What were your feeling responses to the brief reference to the sexuality of ostomates? What do you feel about sexually active people with disabilities? You might like to discuss some of these issues with colleagues or your clinical team if you are caring for older people.

◆ Do you have any thoughts and feelings about active sexuality by people with stomas?

◆ What feelings are aroused in you by the idea of a couple in their 70s making love daily?

◆ How might these feelings inform your practice?

◆ In your practice, how do you acknowledge the fact of continuing sexuality among older people?

◆ Can you give an example of someone you have cared for who is still sexually active in their 70s or older?

◆ What are the implications for care in your own practice from these examples?

In some instances, where there are chronic shortages of staff for instance, or where the flow of patients is so great that recognition of the individual is impeded, the quality of clinical practice is interrupted and disturbed. A gradual erosion of the worker's sense of their own professional self is brought about Sadly, among such pressurised workers, recognition of the patients' individual needs often becomes replaced by the time-saving attitude 'the professional knows best'. This shortcut to thinking and developing relationships with patients seems to occur most frequently when stress levels are at their highest. Management colleagues require information from practitioners if they are to respond adequately and appropriately to the needs of the service. Often, written information alerts more attention.

The manager's task

To achieve a high quality of patient care the manager must ensure adequate resources to provide for staff needs. These should include the provision of funding for continuing training, to include:

- recognised time for further training
- peer clinical discussion groups with support from experienced leaders on site
- reflective practice in a seminar training group.

To focus the work of management, do you keep your manager informed of the needs of your day to day clinical practice? Do you ensure that they understand the work of your team? How can they respond to your needs if they are not kept informed? This is all part of clinical work.

The challenge to the practitioner

The practitioner is challenged to recognise that clinical skills depend not only upon the individual practitioner but also upon the social system and ambience provided by the whole clinical team. The practitioner has responsibility for keeping the line management informed of clinical innovation, to enable recognition and support from them as an integral part of patient care.

Reflection point 3.9

Having read this chapter, has your particular area of clinical expertise received attention? If not, it would be a useful exercise to review the reflection points and consider whether their contents could be addressed to you. Has the chapter been of interest to you? What did you like about it? What seemed difficult? What changes would you have liked?

- If you are already comfortably aware of, and work with, the sexual needs presented to you in practice, it would be useful to remind yourself of the time that you found most difficult and why that was. Write it down and think how you would react today.

- Do you talk about your experiences and help to make other members of your staff team more at ease? Have you considered starting a regular team discussion on the topic of patients' psychosexual needs and sexual care?

- If you are still uncomfortable in addressing these needs with patients, set aside time and write. Set down the worst thing that could happen if you asked a patient how they thought their illness affected their sexual life. Then ask yourself how you would cope with that worst eventuality and write that down. What would you find the most comfortable response? Do you think you could try if you asked someone to mentor your work?

- Do you see the necessity for this work? If so, write what you think makes it so difficult for you to take the initiative with patients. How soon do you think you will be ready and confident to begin this important clinical work?

BIBLIOGRAPHY

The following papers should be readily available from your professional library and should help to stimulate your thinking and discussion about the health care needs of gay and lesbian people.

James T, Harding I, Corbett K 1994 Biased care. Nursing Times 90 (51): 28–30
This paper reports on research into lesbian's and gay men's experiences of nursing care.

Caulfield H, Platzer H 1998 Next of kin. Nursing Standard 13 (7): 47–49
This paper discusses patients' next of kin. Does the term include partners and same-sex partners?

Taylor I, Robertson A 1994 The health needs of gay men: a discussion of the literature and implications for nursing. Journal of Advanced Nursing 20: 560–566
This paper specifically encourages appropriate training about gay issues.

Weeks J, Donovan C, Heaphy B 1996 Families of choice. Patterns of non-heterosexual relationships. South Bank University, London.
An interesting study of single-sex relationships. This book may stimulate you to explore issues about sexuality in relation to particular patients in your care.

REFERENCES

Benner P 1984 From novice to expert: excellence and power in clinical nursing practice. Addison Wesley, Menlo Park, CA
Berne E 1968 Transactional analysis. In: The games people play, Penguin, London, p 29
Caulfield H, Platzer H 1998 Next of kin. Nursing Standard 13(7): 47–49
Casement P 1990 Further learning from the patient. Routledge, London
Cooper E, Guillebaud J 1999 Sexuality and disability: a guide for everyday practice. Radcliffe Medical Press, Oxon
Cort E 1998 Nurses' attitudes to sexuality in caring for cancer patients. Nursing Times 94(42): 54–56
Gillespie-Sells K, Hill M, Robbins B 1998 She dances to different drums. Research into disabled women's sexuality. King's Fund, London
Goffman E 1961 Asylums. Anchor, London
Guardian 1996 Delivery Distress. (15 October)
Huish M, Kumar D, Stones C 1998 Stoma surgery and sexual problems in ostomates. Sexual and Marital Therapy 13(3): 311–328
James T, Harding I, Corbett K 1994 Biased care. Nursing Times 90(51): 28–30
Kafka F 1992 The complete short stories. Minerva, London
Kitzinger J 1990 Recalling the pain. Nursing Times 86(3): 38–40
Moggach D 1995 Changing babies and other short stories. William Heinemann, London
Nightingale F 1859 (new edition 1980) Notes on nursing. Harrison/Churchill Livingstone, London

Penman J 1998 Action research in the care of patients with sexual anxieties. Nursing Standard 13 (13–15): 47–50

Sacks O 1986 A leg to stand on. Pan, London

Savage J 1995 Interaction and embodied knowledge. In: Nursing intimacy, an ethnographic approach to nurse–patient interactions. Scutari, London, pp 67, 68

Schon D A 1987 Teaching artistry through reflection-in-action. In: Educating the reflective practitioner. Jossey Bass, San Francisco

Shepherd B 1994 Patients' views of rehabilitation. Nursing Standard 9(10): 27–30

Taylor I, Robertson A 1994 The health needs of gay men: a discussion of the literature and implications for nursing. Journal of Advanced Nursing 20: 560–566

Waterhouse J, Metcalfe M 1991 Attitudes towards nurses discussing sexual concerns with patients. Journal of Advanced Nursing 16: 1048–1054

Weerakoon P, O'Sullivan V 1998 Inappropriate patient sexual behaviour in physiotherapy practice. Physiotherapy 84(10): 491–499

Winnicott D W 1969 Physiotherapy and human relations In: Winnicott C, Shepherd R, Davis M (eds) 1989 Psychoanalytic explorations. Karnac Books, London

Zilbergeld B 1999 The new male sexuality. Bantam, New York

4

Reflection and the development of skill

Doreen Clifford

KEY ISSUES

◆ The value of the patient as coach

◆ Managing involvement and attachment

◆ Fresh ideas and tolerating not knowing

◆ Balancing thinking and feelings

◆ The hierarchy of feelings that can support or interrupt work

◆ Keeping a reflective diary as an aid to developing practice

INTRODUCTION

In previous chapters the practitioner's awareness of each patient's sexuality has been considered. This chapter moves on to consider how, following this awareness, psychosexual care might be offered and given.

It is taken for granted that interpersonal skills are learnt from interpersonal experiences, therefore a 'how to' guide cannot be written. However, the hope is that this chapter will help in your reflection on how feelings may act as a guide to the interpersonal experiences you have gained when caring for patients' sexual health needs. Once again it is useful to consider the research work, which suggests that many patients wish practitioners would raise issues of sexuality with them (Waterhouse & Metcalfe 1991).

THINKING AND IDEAS

The patient as coach

In some respects the patient can become a guide or coach for the development of psychosexual practice. If the practitioner encourages the patient to lead the conversation then much can be learned from listening to the patient's viewpoint. In this situation the patient's views and feelings are not constrained by the practitioner's framework or questions and practitioners can learn about patients' needs, hopes and fears. It is, however, often helpful for the practitioner to make some enquiry or to encourage the patient to lead the way. When conversations are patient-led the practitioner does not have to be anxious about whether to ask this or that question and the patient's privacy is protected.

The patient-led mode of work is not easy. It is often hard to understand what the patient is indicating, especially when the communication is painful. Therefore practitioners' opportunities for discussion, preferably with colleagues, are important (see Chapter 6, Taking care of the practitioner). Professional discussions may help the practitioner to consider, 'Where was the patient trying to lead me?' and 'What did they want me to know about?' From this, practitioners may progress to defining and refining their skills as, in discussion, they perceive the development of their own practice.

Reflection on practice

Reflection on practice can help in the development of skills and theory. There are many potential benefits, but just three will be highlighted here:

1. To make explicit the knowledge embedded in practice
2. Skill development
3. To think afresh.

Reflection upon practice either alone, or better still with colleagues, gives the opportunity to recognise skills, which are often not acknowledged and are taken for granted. In the describing and laying bare of one's practice, knowledge and expertise are uncovered and may then be recognised and valued. In the light of these recognitions of current skill, opportunities for skill growth and development can often be perceived and acted upon. We need to show both ourselves and others what care is, and that it only becomes visible through talking about it – talking can be particularly fruitful when 'fresh thinking' is encouraged.

Benner (1984) argues in favour of reflection to aid skill development. She observes that 'well charted practices and observations are essential for theory development'. Benner's thinking and descriptions are highly relevant to the development of psychosexual care particularly since she demonstrates how practitioners move into involvement with patients to ensure high standards of clinical care.

Benner describes how clinical knowledge is embedded in the expertise of practice and describes the possibility of practitioner development as follows:

◆ 'the move from reliance on abstract principle to the use of past experience as a standard'
◆ 'then the change to the clinical situation being seen as a complete whole in which only certain parts are relevant'
◆ 'finally the expert practitioner moves from detached observer to involved performer.'

Involvement and attachment

Both Menzies (1960) and Dartington (1993) were concerned that involvement and attachment are viewed as undesirable in hospital hierarchical systems. Discussing her work with student nurses, Dartington suggested there were two important unconscious assumptions prevalent among hospital staff:

◆ 'attachment should be avoided for fear of being overwhelmed with emotional demands that will threaten competence'
◆ 'dependency on colleagues and superiors should be avoided.'

She described how these assumptions inhibit nursing care by creating a fear that 'directness and openness with patients' would lead to attachment and 'impossible demands' from patients. The argument in this book is to the contrary, i.e. the expert practitioner moves from detachment to involvement in skilful health care. It is important to understand that improving the quality of practice requires:

◆ involvement and attachment
◆ recognition of this involvement and the feelings of attachment
◆ study of involvement and feelings of attachment in a supportive group
◆ colleague support.

Making professional skills conscious

Many clinical tasks may appear simple when viewed by an inexperienced observer. However, observations made at this time may 'simultaneously involve intuition and experience' (Savage 1995) and indicate difficulties that require action. An example may be seen in something as simple a recording a blood pressure.

Case study 4.1

In an outpatient clinic a nurse recording a young woman patient's blood pressure noticed that it was raised above that previously recorded. She pointed this out to the patient who said, 'Oh yes, I expect it is. Today I am to have an internal examination by the consultant and I am dreading this.'

The nurse not only recognised that the blood pressure was raised but her openness with the patient enabled her to gain a probable explanation. The patient was able to share her unease and anxiety about the forthcoming procedure which she considered was the reason for her raised blood pressure. Furthermore it gave the opportunity for exploration of her anxiety by the nurse. Not just the technical skill but also the matter of the practitioner 'observing, understanding and acting' (Macleod 1994) moves practice from tasks to skilled work. Note that the practitioner does not necessarily 'understand' completely but asks the patient to engage so that the understanding may be achieved.

Making space for new ideas

Fresh ideas and new knowledge are often painful to acquire, not least because they may require the giving up or modification of long established patterns of understanding. It may seem that well known practices are being devalued. When feeling resistant and resentful of new ideas, it can help to ask oneself whether it is the threat to the comfort provided in well known practice that is unwelcome. Change requires time to put new ideas into practice and to consider and evaluate their validity before incorporating them fully.

Main (1989a), describing the experience of training doctors in psychosexual skills, reports that 'significant changes in attitudes are not usually consolidated until after fifteen to eighteen months of seminar training.' It takes time to achieve new learning and challenges to established attitudes.

Change is emotionally demanding and painful. Taking risks and being prepared to stand for the discomfort of 'not knowing' is part of the learning process. Practising professionals all have their own areas of specialty and skill. For many, however, working with patients' psychosexual realities disturbed by experiences such as illness or hospitalisation is new. This newness demands recognition of the need for fresh ways of thinking to expand practice. In good practice the patient is recognised as a person requiring particular responses, yet to be discovered. Patients frequently express a wish for a practitioner who recognises (knows) this well enough to work alongside them to discover the best way forward. Tolerating 'not knowing' is hard since, as many practitioners admit, until this point their satisfaction has often come from 'knowing' and giving patients the benefits of this knowledge.

The importance of fresh thinking

It can be difficult to think freshly in a situation where one has been working for some time. One valuable way of saving time is by 'knowing' what to do, how to do it and having the ability to respond accurately, sensitively and quickly – a demonstration of embodied knowledge. This ability is important and expected in all patient care. In times of emergency, when there is a need for a speedy response to an event, such knowledge and skill can save pain, morbidity and even lives. Health care practitioners spend a great deal of time training to respond to such events and are valued for their knowledge and response when such skills are required. However, knowledge and skill may also carry a burden – the damage such learning may do to the ability to think freshly in each new relationship with a patient.

Opportunities in developing care offered by fresh thinking

Sometimes a fresh approach can feel like taking risks but the move from 'knowing' into trying a new approach can be rewarding to everyone. We are constantly being alerted to new understandings about the importance of the emotions in health. Cookson (1999) writes of the:

> ...*intimate connection between the brain and the immune system, which explains why your state of mind influences the health of your body. Until recently, scientists had regarded the two as being entirely separate; now they are discovering the molecular pathways that link them.*

It remains for clinicians to recognise that their wish to work in a holistic way with mind and body is supported by such findings.

The argument in this book is that health improves when psychosocial and psychosexual needs are recognised, addressed and are integrated into everyday practice. Parkes & Markus (1998), writing about the implications for care in work with grief, have insights that are also applicable to sexual care:

◆ 'Problems that are ignored seldom go away.'
◆ 'Time spent in creating the secure place in which people feel safe to talk about the unsafe thoughts and feelings that they are experiencing is likely to prevent further problems.'
◆ 'This may well save time in the long run.'

It is possible, for example, to see the relief in a couple when their anxieties about disruptions to their sexuality can be in the open. Such relief from anxiety does not necessarily mean the receipt of good news. For instance, with radical prostatectomy, the news of the likelihood of an impaired sexual response can be devastating. This is especially so when the couple were not prepared in the period before admission for surgery. Care and discussion with someone who will accept and listen to anxious feelings, such as worries about loss of manhood or that a loving partnership will be destroyed, is important. The relief of discussing disrupted feelings can make it possible for a couple to continue talking over their feelings together and to seek understanding and satisfaction in their altered sexual lives.

However, opportunities are sometimes missed. In telling the story of his heart by-pass operation, a middle-aged professional man spoke of the high quality of physical care he had received whilst in hospital. He described how, on many occasions and from different professionals, it had been explained to him exactly what the operation entailed, 'down to the last stitch'. He was, however, surprised that no-one enquired either before or after the operation how he felt about it all – not the physical feelings, but just how it had made him feel. He also noticed that no-one spoke to him about his sexual life. It was only later in a waiting room that he discovered a pamphlet which stated baldly, in one sentence: 'Sexual activity may be resumed after one week' (see Chapter 12).

Reflection point 4.1

Some health care practitioners, recognising the need for information before and following surgical procedures, have written pamphlets and booklets about what a patient may expect before, during and after hospital admission. These have been well received and published by the health authority.

◆ Do you have anything of this kind available to patients in your own sphere of work?

◆ If not, do you consider that it would be useful?

◆ Would you consider working with a colleague and/or a patient to develop such a document, including reference to the likelihood of transitory disturbances to sexual feelings?

◆ Would it include offering opportunities to discuss feelings with staff?

FEELINGS IN DEVELOPING PRACTICE

The value of attachment

Psychosexual care can be an important component during transitions in sexual life; for example, when a young woman is in a transition to becoming actively sexual. The practitioner has opportunities to help or hinder.

Below is an example of an expert practitioner at work. Her work fits the criteria of the expert as described by Benner (1984).

◆ She is experienced.
◆ She compiles information and seeks the relevant parts.
◆ She moves from detached observer to involved performer, 'then things changed' she reports. 'We became like two mature women discussing what to do.'

Case study 4.2

'The young woman came into the clinic. She appeared both young and vulnerable, perhaps about 14, I thought. She was shy, timid, hesitant and I was surprised when she told me that she had just had her sixteenth birthday and was ready to go on the pill.

'I indicated my interest and she told me how she had known her boyfriend for 2 years. They had decided to wait until she was 16 before making love.

'At first I thought, "This is him and his needs," but as I listened it become apparent that the demand was from her. She was determined. This hesitant little girl!

'We started where she was. It was when I asked about her boyfriend and discussed his part in this decision, that things began to change. I took her history and as I touched her to record her blood pressure, our relationship changed. It became like two mature women discussing what might be the best thing to do.

'We had an amazing talk. She listened carefully to the facts I gave her. I talked about looking after herself, of taking care. She asked me questions and we discussed the options open to her.

'As she left she looked like a young woman rather than the little girl who had arrived; she was confident, mature and somehow sure of herself. Something real had changed for her during our meeting, something that allowed her to grow.'

There were so many choices. The practitioner could have indicated disapproval or difficulty about the young woman's decision to use contraception in a number of ways. She could have taken the role of the older expert giving good advice and kindness as to a child. The actions the practitioner chose, however, allowed the young woman to demonstrate her ability to be mature in a co-equal and adult relationship, and indicate her 'growth' on leaving. We can note how the practitioner's feelings changed from rather parental to a co-equal willingness to accept and work with the patient

When reviewing the examples given in this and previous chapters, some of the skills which may be observed as embedded in the practitioner's practice might be defined as:

◆ observation of the presenting patient
◆ recognition of any distress or uncertainty
◆ opportunity given to explore together with the patient
◆ willingness to discuss feelings
◆ involvement in the feelings evoked by the distress
◆ use of the feelings to gain closer contact and aid the situation.

Exploration of unexpected anxieties arising in the practitioner–patient relationship

One difficulty frequently expressed is that of wondering if the opening up of painful topics by the health care practitioner can cause damage for the patient. The following case from an experienced practitioner illustrates how unexpected feelings can enter a clinical situation.

From this story we can observe:

◆ The question asked was from a sexual history pro forma used regularly with new patients
◆ The practitioner had asked the same question on many previous occasions and had considered this to be a routine matter
◆ The response took her completely by surprise
◆ The pain of the response paralysed the practitioner and inhibited the continuation of the work with this patient.

Case study 4.3

The practitioner was taking a sexual history from a new client and during the course of this asked, 'When did you first have sexual intercourse?' a question required by the formal history she was taking. The client, an apparently self-contained and charming young person keen for contraceptive help, dissolved into tears. Through her tears she said she was surprised at her own reaction, but went on to tell of being regularly sexually abused by her uncle from the age of 9 until leaving home. The nurse, listening sympathetically, felt shocked, enraged on the client's behalf and helpless. She expressed her sympathy and concern but felt unable to pursue the story further or attempt to understand the implications for the current sexual relationship.

The practitioner spoke about this to no-one, but some years later, in the course of a psychosexual discussion seminar with a group of colleagues, she told the story. She explained that her chief anxiety was that she may have caused the client damage by her question. She felt the client's tears were her fault and that such a question was too traumatic for the young woman, perhaps causing her more emotional damage and further pain.

During the discussion that followed, a colleague said, 'It was not you who damaged the patient, but her uncle.' This observation seemed of real importance for the practitioner telling the story and led to further discussion. As the discussion continued it was suggested that sensitivity to the client's current situation had been avoided. An opportunity for her to think with the practitioner about the relationship for which she was seeking contraceptive help might have been useful in the light of her disturbing story. It would have allowed focussed sexual health care to continue. However, this was made impossible by the defences alerted in the worker by her identification with the client's distress.

The event described by the patient was so painful that it became unspeakable until it was remembered and resurrected in a place deemed safe enough to talk about it – for both client and nurse! The client felt safe enough to speak with the nurse in the clinic, the nurse felt safe enough to share her experience with colleagues several years after the event.

The question of painful memories arising unexpectedly is of concern to all who work closely with people. Note that the pain the nurse experienced was potentially of value, it gave her a glimpse of the patient's feelings of distress. When this can be understood and respected, the response to the patient can be between two adult people interested in understanding the meaning of the memory for today's purposes, in this case seeking contraception.

The questions raised by this story are legion. Its relevance to your own clinical situation is important. How do you care for both the client and yourself, the practitioner, when painful stories and revelations occur?

Valuing the difference between thinking and feeling

Sometimes we get muddled about thinking and feeling, which are very different. We can 'take' thought, but feelings seem to be involuntary and often appear irrational or confusing, i.e. we become aware of how we feel. Feelings are not always welcome. Sometimes they prove to be unwanted interference in our daily lives. There is no help for it, we feel! What a good thing this is. There is so much about the practitioner–patient relationship we can learn from the study of our feelings at the time.

Reflection point 4.2

There is little doubt that some revelations heard in the practitioner–client relationship make severe demands upon the practitioner. There are many questions that require thought regarding painful events recalled and revealed whilst working with a patient.

When considering your own practice, you may care to make some notes on the following questions:

◆ How might a difficult story be acknowledged at the time with the patient?

◆ Can the practitioner or the patient understand why the story should be recalled on this occasion?

◆ Who should the practitioner discuss this with today?

Reflection point 4.3

Each of us will be aware of events and stories that may have caused us embarrassment, discomfort, difficulty and distress. It is not only what happens to us but how we choose to learn from it that matters. In discussion with a small group of colleagues, reflect on the following questions:

◆ Am I brave enough to talk this over with colleagues?

◆ What am I afraid could happen if I discuss this; for example, am I uncomfortable/self-critical about the way I dealt with it at the time?

◆ Do I fear that confidentiality will not be respected? How can this be agreed within the group?

◆ Can a discussion of this kind expand the clinical skills of each of us in the discussion group?

Reflection point 4.4

It is important to write personal accounts of difficult situations to give you an opportunity to recall the event whilst fresh in your mind (see Keeping a reflective diary, later in Chapter 4).

For this to be an opportunity to expand practice, you should set aside some time for yourself. It will be important to reflect upon what happened, what you did at the time, your actions, your reactions and your feelings both at the time and since the event. Review whether your feelings were uncomfortable, whether you believe that such feelings are not what you should experience. In time it will be possible to find an individual or a group you trust, have confidence in and can think with. It is important to find someone with whom you can discuss your impressions of the situation and who will understand. Suggestions for the notes you could make:

◆ How you worked with the patient on disturbance to their sexual feelings.

◆ What happened between you, how you felt on this occasion.

◆ Do you understand why you feel as you do?

◆ Did you enquire about how the patient was feeling?

◆ Has this proved an opportunity to develop your clinical practice?

Notes for clinical managers

Caring for clinical staff

The development and support of sexual health care depends upon the clinical team managers of nurses, midwives, health visitors, physiotherapists and all others having a responsibility for standards and quality of clinical care. The development and support of sexual health care is dependent on clinical managers recognising and managing staff needs for continuing support.

Box 4.1 Points for manager's reflections

◆ How do I best support the continuing appreciation of the disruption to patients' sexual feelings inherent in the clinical work?

◆ How could I arrange regular opportunities for staff group discussions when things are difficult in this clinical area?

◆ Should I consider organising regular review sessions when staff come to the end of their shift? Such things as: 'How has it been for you today?' or 'Has there been anything you would like to talk over before you leave?' might be useful.

◆ What support do you yourself have from your own manager? Have you considered requesting further training in psychosexual care?

In addition, some feelings are more welcome than others, and are easier to acknowledge to oneself as being worthy and of producing feelings of comfort and satisfaction in the practitioner. It is not easy to like every patient and dislike, if not faced and understood, can inhibit care.

Opportunities and difficulties in working with feelings

For each person there seem to be occasions when some feelings are more acceptable than others. When the practitioner is tired, for example, the client

---

Case study 4.4

During a group discussion, one ward sister told the story of two patients in her ward suffering from severe bronchial illnesses. One was quiet, undemanding, very aware of the efforts made on her behalf by the staff and spoke warmly to her relatives of her gratitude for the standard of care she received.

The other patient, whom we will call Mrs H, was described as a 'hypochondriac' – always complaining about her illness. She made constant demands for attention which seldom seemed to please her, being either too slow or insufficient for her needs. She received larger doses of medication because she complained so much about her illness.

During discussion it emerged that Mrs H was disliked and rather avoided by the staff on the ward. In other words, the label 'hypochondriac' was used to avoid mentioning how difficult it was to like this patient. However, when the discussion reached these conclusions, something surprising happened. The ward sister concerned developed an interest in this 'hypochondriacal' patient. She returned to her work determined to get to know Mrs H better.

is likely to receive less focussed attention. When the practitioner is already preoccupied by concerns of any nature, there is little ability to remain alert to the presentation of distress.

Read the case study of Mrs H described above. In a subsequent meeting, the ward sister reported that she had spent time trying to improve her relationship with Mrs H, although she was a difficult person and remained hard to like. However, the effect of her attention had been that the woman began to be less demanding and became slightly more appreciative of the care she was receiving. She therefore became easier to look after. Both patients recovered and were discharged on the same day.

Another approach would have been to see the difficulty experienced by staff and their dislike of the patient as part of Mrs H's assessment, to be put in the care plan and explored. Instead the staff were ashamed of not liking her, then labelled Mrs H, thus excusing their feelings. It was when the feelings were faced squarely that Mrs H was given attention, the difficulties in caring for her were faced and she began to be more acceptable.

Many of us have similar experiences in our own work. There are some feelings about patients and clients that we find more acceptable than others. Whereas comfortable feelings fitting with our notions of good practice are acceptable, other feelings not fitting this 'ideal' are denied. This situation is so commonplace as to seem unremarkable, but when these uncomfortable feelings are denied the patient is in danger of missing out on some important aspects of care. If we can recognise that difficult feelings are interesting and worthy of study there is opportunity to improve our strategies for care, as occurred with Mrs H.

Feelings can provoke moral judgements in the practitioner

Working with feelings is interesting – nothing should be taken at face value and every feeling deserves thought. Sometimes it is as though moral judgements are made about feelings considered good and others that appear less than worthy. However, it is not easy to control our feelings, so we should not feel shame when they are not as we expect them to be. Yet we tend to make severe criticisms of ourselves for having feelings we judge unworthy or unhelpful in relation to clients.

It is interesting to note the difficulty of recognising feelings that fail to meet the high clinical standards we set ourselves. Unrecognised in oneself, difficult feelings can inhibit broader understandings in the practitioner– patient couple and limit the care offered (seen in the example of the responses to Mrs H).

Some practitioners find it useful to take a moment to think about something they feel:

'I feel rather critical of this woman. I do not like this feeling. How interesting...'

'Is this *my* feeling and if so why?'

'Perhaps it is also *her* feeling that I am reflecting in myself...'

'Let me try to find out.'

The practitioner may then ask the client:

'I wonder how this leaves you feeling, a bit uncomfortable perhaps? Would you like to talk it over with me?'

The practitioner:

◆ recognises discomfort in self
◆ examines those feelings
◆ thinks about the findings
◆ offers some of this recognition for consideration with the patient.

Recognising a hierarchy of morality in feelings

Practitioners who have studied their emotional responses to patients for many years are clear that recognition of feelings is the key to skill development. Professionals are individuals too and each person appears to find some feelings more or less acceptable. Feelings such as compassion, kindness and concern are usually well regarded. Negative feelings make demands on both recognition and tolerance and yet are potential assets in understanding how the patient feels.

Some factors, such as the maintenance of severe self-critical attitudes about the professional self, may interfere with developing new skills. (You may recognise this in a colleague who denies that they ever feel impatience or irritation with a patient.)

One of the concepts developed in psychosexual seminars is that the professional can prove to be a different practitioner with different patients and that it helps to study how this comes about. The question, 'What kind of practitioner did *this* patient have today?' can reveal hidden information about the relationship between the two and how they have reacted upon each other. More than just an interesting idea, it provides opportunity to develop understanding of both the patient's feelings and how to make an appropriate response. Requiring the ability to think upon one's feet, Schon (1987) describes this work as 'reflection in action', enabling recognition and response *at the time* to feelings evoked by an individual patient. The understanding that responses are unique to each relationship and can be used to develop the joint work of understanding with the patient is something that the reader can test for themselves.

There is a skilled technique of studying the practitioner–patient relationship to understand how a patient is feeling and to learn more of their concerns.

◆ Did my patient have a kindly practitioner or an irritable one? The answer may be a clue to how the patient was feeling on this occasion.
◆ Test the situation by asking a neutral question indicating interest, such as, 'How are you feeling today?', allowing the patient to reveal a particular concern or worry that is disturbing them, or just share the fact that they feel 'out of sorts', making them feel irritable perhaps.

Some of this apparently simple response by the practitioner is dependent upon two things:

1. The practitioner being prepared to acknowledge uncomfortable feelings like irritation within the professional self.
2. The practitioner regarding such feelings as valid information.

A fresh view into practice can be opened when feelings can be recognised as tools in understanding.

As already suggested in this chapter, not all feelings are acceptable all of the time. Some practitioners find certain feelings within themselves quite unacceptable. The best that can be asked is that our ideas do not remain static but are scrutinised regularly with the aid of reflection in a group, by keeping a reflective diary or in supervision. Nevertheless, it is important that we examine the subjective feelings arising during work with patients. Examination at the time gives us an opportunity to fine tune our responses to the patients' psychosexual needs and allows the work and focus of the practitioner–patient relationship to continue.

Case study 4.5

In a seminar discussion group, an experienced worker sympathetically described a patient seeking contraceptive advice. Despite this specialist practitioner spending time talking the patient through the wide variety of methods available the woman could find nothing to suit her. The practitioner felt that she had somehow failed the woman. During the seminar discussion it became apparent to the other group members that the practitioner had become irritated with the patient. The practitioner had not recognised her irritation at the time. The avoidance of uncomfortable feelings meant that there was no attempt to understand the possible meaning of the patient's lack of satisfaction in the consultation. Consequently, the woman received no help in exploring why she could find nothing acceptable. Whether the patient's lack of satisfaction reflected a missing feeling about herself, her sexual feelings, or the relationship with her partner, we cannot know. We can, however, recognise that practitioner–patient work stopped when the practitioner's feelings of irritation at the lack of satisfaction/suitability were not acknowledged.

Why work stops

When unwanted or unwished for feelings go unrecognised, work between patient and practitioner stops.

In the above case, the practitioner's liking for the patient disrupted her ability to empathise with the patient's feelings of difficulty and failure. The practitioner merely took on these feelings as her own. Handled differently, recognition of irritation could have given her food for thought and enabled a different and more helpful outcome.

A SUGGESTED HIERARCHY OF FEELINGS THAT CAN SUPPORT OR INTERRUPT WORK

A list of feelings has been recognised and studied during psychosexual seminars as those which frequently provoke difficulties. Because some feelings are more acceptable to practitioner and patient than others, this does not mean that they are necessarily easier to work with. Remember that 'liking' interrupted the work in the above case.

The feelings are set into three groups (Box 4.2). Some seem to be commonly recognised as acceptable, others are presented as difficult, while some are hard to recognise and accept. Patients also contribute their willingness or not to recognise painful or difficult feelings within themselves and whether they wish to discuss them with the practitioner.

Box 4.2 highlights an incomplete and constantly changing list, and the reader will have ideas and contributions from practice which will provide new avenues to be explored. It is possible to view this list of feelings as receiving pressure from both patient and practitioner, changing the possibility of accepting and working with some feelings.

Practitioner → Feeling ← Patient

The practitioner and patient both contribute to what is or is not acceptable. Chapter 6 explores the concept of the projection of difficult feelings into and by the practitioner and there is a recognition of the way that some feelings may be denied by the practitioner.

Theory is composed of ever changing and developing understandings. Your own thinking, reflections and practice have a great deal to contribute to the furtherance of such understandings.

Defences against pain in the practitioner

We can see from both experience and Box 4.2 that some feelings cause distress in particular people, whether patient or practitioner. Pain is to be respected and cared for: in the practitioner by continuing training in skill development, and in the patient by the professional clinical team.

Box 4.2 Feelings that can provoke difficulty in psychosexual care

Acceptable feelings
- ◆ Liking a patient
- ◆ Feeling sorry for (pity)
- ◆ Compassion
- ◆ Identification with patient's difficulty
- ◆ Some feelings evoked by tears (e.g. compassion, sympathy)

Difficult feelings
- ◆ Disconnection
- ◆ Contempt
- ◆ Uncertainty
- ◆ Not knowing
- ◆ Feeling at a loss
- ◆ Helplessness
- ◆ Confusion (Note: this feeling can also be an occasion for avoiding work)
- ◆ Dislike
- ◆ Embarrassment
- ◆ Irritation
- ◆ Feelings evoked by tears (e.g. withdrawal, insincere response, irritation, disbelief)

Unacceptable (i.e. unrecognised) feelings
- ◆ Fear
- ◆ Dislike
- ◆ Contempt
- ◆ Anger
- ◆ Distaste
- ◆ Disgust
- ◆ Hatred.

Main (1989b) writes about the recognition of feelings experienced and sometimes defended against by practitioners in this work.

The trained disciplined use of subjectivity as a source of scientific information is rare; moreover, it will inevitably often involve us in pain. We need not be surprised therefore, and none of us can afford to be critical, if (practitioners) seek ways of limiting their subjectivity and of alleviating the strains of uncomfortably close encounters; if they distance themselves from patients' distress in various ways ... But if we dare value subjectivity then we may come to legitimize the study of the subjective feelings of (practitioners), the ways they at present are ignored in unconscious and undisciplined ways and how they can be used in deliberate and disciplined fashion to throw light on the patient and his problems. (pp. 213–216)

There seem to be two kinds of defensiveness in practice:

1. Those defences necessary for function: for example, when working in theatre or ITU, identification with the patient would mean inability to use all the physical skills required in this work.
2. Those which interrupt function, i.e. when the practitioner is troubled, leading to failure to recognise that colleagues and patients also have feelings. (An example is when a patient's pain alerts pain from a similar experience in the practitioner's own life (see Chapter 6)).

Reflection point 4.5

Do you recognise any of the hierarchy of feelings listed above from your own practice? Do you recognise the defences against involvement with patients described?

How would your list of acceptable and difficult feelings read?

You might like to make notes on three patients you work with; in relation to these patients what feelings have you experienced? Allocate these feelings to three categories:

◆ acceptable
◆ difficult
◆ unacceptable.

Does this thinking give you ideas about alternative ways of approaching these feelings? Can you see any ways forward in your practice by reflecting in this way?

Can you remember and describe the last encounter with a patient where you were not able to respond as you would wish because of your difficult feelings? What feelings were those?

Having completed this exercise alone, encourage a few colleagues to undertake it. In discussion together, try to clarify whether such thinking could inform your practice and enlarge your skills in sexual health care.

Issues that may inhibit continuing work with feelings

Work with sexual health issues alerts practitioners to difficulties with the feelings experienced by both themselves and their patients. There is no doubt that the ability to continue to work with particular feelings differs from day to day and from person to person. Some feelings in the practitioner can interfere in the work of care:

◆ feeling tired
◆ being in a new situation
◆ being under strain, shorthanded, running late
◆ personal distress, e.g. bereavement
◆ feeling unsupported, perhaps criticised, in the clinical situation.

It is important that we accept our own feelings on such occasions, freeing us to continue working and remain 'available' to the patients' needs. Perhaps the standards set by the practitioner are impossibly high. If we are to be alert to our perception of patients' feelings, we need to recognise our own needs and be aware of particularly vulnerable times in our practice.

A practitioner, feeling very stressed by the events of the day, should be confident enough to say to a patient, 'I am sorry but this is not a good time for us to discuss this matter. I am not at my best. Could we arrange to meet again in the next few days when I will have time and space to talk this over properly with you?' A patient receiving respect in this way is likely to have a positive feeling about continuing work with this practitioner.

By continuing reflection with colleagues the practitioner can become aware of the ordinary defences preventing the recognition of difficult feelings and can remain alert to them.

KEEPING A REGULAR REFLECTIVE DIARY

Earlier in the chapter, the effects of reflection upon practice were considered as helping in the development of skills and the integration of theory. In turn, practitioners can contribute to theory by keeping a careful record of their reflections and being willing to contribute their conclusions and developments made in association with others.

The three potential benefits highlighted earlier and repeated here are:

◆ To make explicit the knowledge embedded in practice
◆ Skill development
◆ To think afresh.

Keeping a reflective diary is a useful way of keeping oneself aware of developing skills and any difficulties that may impede their use in practice. This chapter has been considering the importance of developing and maintaining standards of practice, and discussing, comparing and reflecting upon practice with colleagues as a way of developing skills. Another useful way of making opportunity to reflect upon and enhance practice is by keeping a 'reflective diary'.

A diary is personal and private, and should be an account of patients you meet with psychosexual difficulties, your reflections on the encounter and what you learned from that interpersonal event. It is useful to consider whether you felt content with the work you did. In a private diary there is opportunity to be open with oneself so that any judgements on your actions are your own. You have no need to impress anyone with your knowledge or abilities but can take time to consider the practitioner–patient encounter and the possibilities of growing further skills. It is an opportunity to describe and reflect on your handling of an encounter and the part feelings had to play in your responses (Box 4.3).

Some observations you might make are:

◆ What did you feel about the patient? Was the feeling comfortable or not?
◆ When did you recognise the feeling? Did you use it in the work; if so, how?
◆ Did the feeling change during the encounter?
◆ Were you able to enrol the patient in the study of their feelings as an aid to you both understanding the difficulties under discussion?

The actual writing of the diary gives you the time and discipline for reflection and an opportunity to think about what you have learned from the encounter that will alert you or make you more available when next you recognise your feelings. Perhaps, because the diary is private, you will be able to be more open and demanding of yourself when writing reflections on your work.

Box 4.3 Sample reflective diary questions

Example: perhaps you felt irritated on a particular occasion.

◆ What effect did this feeling have upon your work?
◆ Did the irritation force you to retreat from the patient or become impatient in your response to them?
◆ Did you become insincerely nice, perhaps because of your discomfort when you realised your feelings of irritation?
◆ Were you able to ascertain whether the irritation 'came in with' the patient; was it perhaps something left over in you from a previous encounter?
◆ Were you able to recognise the irritation thoughtfully at the time and, thinking on your feet, see that the feeling gave you a focus for work?

More than likely you missed it and only afterwards, thinking about the practitioner–patient encounter, did you realise what had happened.

The important thing is to recognise feelings. Initially these understandings may come afterwards as you think over and write about them. With practice, you will recognise them at the time, thus making them available to become a helpful tool for your work since they may be a version of the patient's experience.

Remember the purpose of this account is to demonstrate to yourself the progress you are making in developing skills in psychosexual health care. This can be of particular benefit when sharing such events in a discussion group with colleagues who are similarly attempting to develop their skills in this work.

CONCLUSION

This chapter considered how change can be a difficult experience but may also prove a learning opportunity for the practitioner. It addresses the demands that working with feelings makes upon the practitioner in relation to both clinical staff and their managers. Attention has been drawn to the importance of recognising and managing staff needs for continuing support in this difficult area of work.

The different ways in which reflection can guide understanding of interpersonal experiences when caring for patients' sexual health needs have been demonstrated. When there are opportunities for such reflection practitioners can develop skills to recognise and respond appropriately to their patients' needs for sexual care. Without this, holistic care is not possible, but practitioners who have gained some skills in sexual care are rewarded. Many have spoken of an increased sense of their professional selves and greater confidence about working with future patients.

BIBLIOGRAPHY

There is a great deal published about reflective practice – these are some recommendations you may find accessible and stimulating.

Macleod M 1994 It's the little things that count: the hidden complexity of everyday clinical nursing practice. Journal of Clinical Nursing 3: 361–368
This is a study of everyday experience in nursing and how it contributes to the development of expertise.

Marland G, McSherry W 1997 The reflective diary: an aid to practice-based learning. Nursing Standard 12(13–15): 49–52
The authors describe a small study for the development and use of reflective diaries.

Schon D A 1987 Educating the reflective practitioner. Jossey Bass, San Francisco
For deeper reading Chapter 2, Teaching Artistry through Reflection-in-action, is recommended.

REFERENCES

Benner P 1984 From novice to expert: excellence and power in clinical nursing practice. Addison Wesley, Menlo Park, CA, Ch 1, p 2; Ch 2, p 13

Cookson C 1999 On the alert for cries of pain. *Financial Times* (13/14 February), Weekend, p ii

Dartington A 1993 Where angels fear to tread. Idealism, despondency and inhibition in thought in hospital nursing. Winnicott Studies (Spring): 21–41

Macleod M 1994 It's the little things that count: the hidden complexity of everyday clinical nursing practice. Journal of Clinical Nursing 3: 361–368

Main T F 1989a Training for the acquisition of knowledge or the development of skill? In: Johns J (ed) The ailment and other psychoanalytic essays. Free Association Press, London, p 230

Main T F 1989b Some medical defences against anxiety. In: Johns J (ed) The ailment and other psychoanalytic essays. Free Association Press, London, pp 213–214

Menzies I E P 1960 A case study in the functioning of social systems against anxiety. Human Relations 13(2): 95–121

Parkes C M, Markus A 1998 Coping with loss. BMJ Publications, London, pp 81–89

Savage J 1995 Nursing intimacy, an ethnographic approach to nurse–patient interactions. Scutari, London, p 67

Schon D A 1987 Teaching artistry through reflection-in-action. In: Educating the reflective practitioner. Jossey Bass, San Francisco

Waterhouse J, Metcalfe M 1991 Attitudes towards nurses discussing sexual concerns with patients. Journal of Advanced Nursing 16: 1048–1054

5

Caring for sexuality in loss

Doreen Clifford

KEY ISSUES

◆ How a variety of losses disrupt feelings about self and sexual function

◆ The help patients may be seeking

◆ Developing further skills in helping with sexuality

◆ Caring for the distress of loss brought about by treatment

◆ Continuing care for grief and loss in aiding recovery or facing alternatives

◆ Helping with some resolution of grieving

INTRODUCTION

A sense of loss is a common feeling throughout life from the first sense of being alone as an infant to the sense of loneliness that old age can bring. This chapter discusses loss as one of the stimuli to sexual distress. A sense of loss may be stimulated by many experiences, including the death of someone dear, ill health and childbirth. Loss can be experienced following surgical intervention, medical treatments and neurological conditions. Practitioners' alertness to patients' feelings of loss can help the return to a sense of an integrated and sexual self.

This chapter considers the effects that loss has upon the way people experience themselves, their relationships and their sexual lives. It does not attempt to address personal bereavement at the loss of loved ones which is followed by grief and mourning. Loss is explored here as the experience during and following illness, chronic disease, surgery and other conditions that change perceptions of the self. Parkes & Markus (1998) suggest that:

Though the grief which follows physical losses is different from the griefs which follow loss of a person, there are important similarities, and these situations teach us much about the process of adaptation which comes into play whenever one set of habitual assumptions must be abandoned and a new set learned.

Caring for sexuality includes recognising and understanding how the experience of loss can often change the image of the self. Feelings play a part in the maintenance of self and sexuality, and understanding this is important to the continuing development of skilled practice.

In the description of her own work with grief in families, Pincus (1997) wrote, 'how many symptoms of physical or mental disturbance are caused by unrecognised repressed grief for the loss of an important person?' It is suggested here that unrecognised grief may also relate to losses within the self and sexual partnership.

Chapter 4 considered the way that change can be a learning situation for the practitioner. The experience of giving up established ideas was suggested as necessary for the integration of fresh ideas and developing new skills. This chapter suggests that the pain of grief, when integrated into the personality, also offers opportunities for growth. Parkes & Markus (1998) believe that 'there is evidence that handled right losses can foster maturity and personal growth.'

Loss as a cause for grief and distress

Loss of any kind means a disturbance to the sense of self and to feelings of well-being, feelings that are implicit in each person's sense of themselves and therefore their sexuality. Loss can impair the ability to maintain relationships in the face of the pain it incurs because the focus of feelings turns to the self and there is a retreat from relationships with others. The loss easily overlooked is the one health care professionals meet most often, simply the loss of health.

To some extent the feelings following bereavement (Pincus 1997) described below are experienced with every significant loss, including health:

◆ shock – 'We might notice that for physical shock recommendations are warmth and rest. Instead, keeping busy and denial tend to happen'
◆ a controlled phase – 'arrangements to be made, funeral faced and endured'
◆ restlessness/pining/searching for the lost person
◆ sadness/anger/hostility
◆ regression alternating with maturity and self-discipline.

When the worker offers attention to feelings of loss, recognising that they will affect the patient's life, then many people suffering ill health can be offered help to recover from their effects. The converse is also true. Ignoring the feelings of ill people fails to help. Mrs Anderson's story highlights a disappointing experience by someone suffering a chronic illness. It is also possible to follow the way that the feelings described in this story mirror Pincus's suggestions.

Case study 5.1

Mrs Anderson is a woman of 60. Until the onset of arachnoiditis, she was fully active, involved in her community and with her family. She especially loved playing on the floor with her small grandchildren and sharing in their fun and physical care. With her loss of health came the realisation that she must curtail many of her former activities. It became necessary to withdraw from most of her community responsibilities. Within the family she found that even to stretch down to pick up a baby or toddler caused her a great deal of pain which might incapacitate her for days. The loss of community commitments, along with her other losses of close and loving physical contact with the children of the family, left her feeling angry and sad. She spent time and energy searching for information about her illness; contacting appropriate groups, searching the Internet and reading as much information as she could find. She continually hoped that there was a 'cure' or at least a treatment which might allow her to continue with her life as formerly. When this search failed her, it left her grieving for all that she experienced as loss, including the sense of herself as a useful person. She found herself feeling self-critical at times and alert to any hint from others that they might consider her 'lazy' or unhelpful. Her considerable insight into this did not prevent feelings of grief for all she had lost along with her health. Slowly, she adapted to her new situation and found different ways to be of service in her community.

Months later, her feelings of anger still surprise her at times, especially when triggered by health care workers who cannot seem to understand her and appear uncaring about her damaged life.

Mrs Anderson has not been invited to speak about her life changes by any health care professional that she has met in outpatient, X-ray, physiotherapy, pain clinic or other departments and she has not volunteered to any professional just how she feels. Her experiences lead her to believe that the practitioners have no interest in how her life is affected by her condition. No-one has ever enquired about the effect upon her sexual life of this disabling condition, so she does not feel entitled to raise the issue with anyone. She usually meets helpful and busy workers, who get on with their care for her body. She does not believe that they are unfeeling, but apparently see their role as confined to her physical care. She often leaves such sessions feeling less than herself. She has described how she feels as 'low', 'sad' and 'guilty' for having expected a different help from the practitioners who in other respects she values.

Reflection point 5.1

It is possible to follow Pincus's description of the course of grief through Mrs Anderson's story. Are you aware of a similar theme running through the life of someone in your care at present? Would it help your work with them to discuss:

◆ How they consider that their illness has affected their life?

◆ Whether and how feelings about their sexual self are disturbed by their experiences.

◆ If they have enough information about the possible future course of the illness.

◆ What practical advice they would value.

Disruption to sexual function can become a significant loss for anyone affected, and may be the cause of misery, disharmony in a couple and profound unhappiness. Such grief deserves to be properly addressed by the practitioner. When the results of surgery and radiotherapy, for example, are unalterable and drugs cannot be changed, then it is imperative that opportunity to discuss the effect upon the person's life is given. The practitioner should be prepared to discuss feelings with the patient or couple, along with suggestions and ideas for alternative sexual sharing in their partnership.

Case study 5.2

In an oncology department a practitioner asked a woman outpatient whether everything was alright sexually. Her reply was, 'I am so grateful to you. Eleven years; eleven bloody years since my treatment began and this is the first time anyone has mentioned sex to me. Because of the difficulties I had after treatment, my first marriage ended in divorce. There was no-one I could talk to, I didn't know where to turn. Now I have a new partner and I would like to talk to you about this' ... and she did.

This story underlines that patients frequently need help during and following treatment, and value practitioners who are willing to discuss any sexual difficulties arising.

Penetrative intercourse is not the only way for a couple to demonstrate their love and to excite and satisfy each other. Some people find the tactility of the skin, oiled and massaged by their partner, stimulating and enjoyable, whilst others can discover the shared pleasures of oral sex. Kissing, tender touching and explorations of other areas of sensitivity can bring a sense of worth back into a loving relationship. It is important to encourage exploration between partners for them to make discoveries of different ways of loving.

Practitioners may find it helpful to contact SPOD, 286 Camden Road, London N7 OBJ, UK, Telephone 0207 607 8851. A resource pack is on offer which includes information leaflets on such subjects as:

◆ sex after stroke
◆ sex after heart attack
◆ incontinence and sex
◆ a sex education video for young people with physical disabilities.

Some effects of expanding practice to address feelings

There is evidence (e.g. Kaplan et al 1989) to suggest that when the practitioner recognises distress and enquires about how the patient's life has been affected by ill health there is a marked effect on recovery. A lively example is seen in Macklin et al's (1983) report on research into dyspnoea with a multi-professional team. They discuss a project in which a group of patients who received help from psychotherapists, doctors and others were assessed for the effectiveness of different practice. The practitioner found to be most effective in improving this distressing condition was the nurse. She talked with her patients about how they managed their lives with this disabling symptom and explored their problems. She offered practical advice and discussed medical treatment. Patients who received this psychosocial nursing care experienced sustained relief of their dyspnoea (see Chapter 12).

The help patients seek with loss of health

The apparent simplicity of this approach is reassuring. In discussion with patients, it seems that the requirement of many is a desire for:

◆ the expression of concern and interest for them as individuals
◆ opportunity to discuss and explore the feelings provoked in them by their illness
◆ how their illness/condition affects feelings about their sexual selves
◆ discussion on the effects that ill health has upon their lives and families
◆ practical advice and opportunity to discuss the course of their condition
◆ opportunity to hear more about the likely course of their condition.

Practitioner expectations

Practitioners often tend to believe that they are required to be experts with ready answers – an expectation that may lead to uncertainty. In seminar discussions many practitioners have admitted that feelings of uncertainty impel them to keep giving bodily care even when they know psychosocial care is required. When this happens, both patient and practitioner are disappointed. However, those practitioners who are able to maintain emotional contact and attachment with the patient and their feelings, seem to gain more satisfaction from their work. Discussion with patients as an integral part of care does not need to extend the time allotted to treatment.

There is evidence that distress caused by loss of health is often demonstrated in everyday clinical work but remains for the most part unrecognised by practitioners. Slow healing – for example, irritability, grumbling, solitariness, a shallow brightness – can mask feelings. Each individual will perceive illness and show distress in their own way. A marked effect on recovery would be observed if practitioners addressed this distress with patients, enquiring about the effect their loss of health has had upon their lives. Recognising the patient's whole self following mourning for the loss of self-image can lead to an integration of feelings, improved perception of self and sense of worth. Many believe that this in turn leads to an enhanced immune system, which aids the recovery of health (Cookson 1999).

Developing further skills in helping with sexuality

The words we use

Our culture does not assist us much in acquiring a language of ordinary sexuality. Despite the new openness about sex, the words commonly used are guarded and the actual naming of parts, particularly female genitals, is still taboo except sometimes among close friends.

Gloria Steinem (1998), describing the way that the 'well educated, strong and informed women' of her family referred to female genitalia, writes: 'I come from the "down there" generation. That is, those were the words – spoken rarely and in a hushed voice – that the women in my family used to refer to all female genitalia, internal or external … it was not that they were ignorant of terms like vagina, vulva or clitoris and they were neither unliberated nor straight laced', but she did not hear words that were accurate, let alone proud, when speaking of female genitals.

Many practitioners have also referred to 'not knowing the right way to speak' and 'not knowing the words'. When this is so among professional health workers, we should be alerted to the difficulties some patients have in finding the words to ask us to understand their situation about disturbances in physical and emotional sexuality.

If patients use vague terms such as 'down there' the practitioner may be in a dilemma. She can either continue with the phrase 'down there', or use words such as vulva, labia and clitoris which may make the patient feel uncomfortable. The words may sound medical and distant to the patient, or the patient may not know exactly what they mean. The practitioner may need to teach the patient, negotiating about words and their meaning. Some practitioners find a pelvic model and a hand mirror useful in locating the parts under discussion with the patient.

Some conditions and diseases are seen so frequently by health care practitioners that it is difficult to remember that for some individuals they represent either a new experience or the continuation of a long-standing one. It is tempting, when short of time and under pressure of work, not to pay attention to the individual but rather to hurry on through an outpatient or treatment clinic.

Reflection point 5.2

Stop for a moment to consider these examples of familiar disabilities met in practice. Consider whether, addressing the feelings of an individual, you might affect their quality of life.

◆ What might be the effect of a sports injury to knee or groin upon the perceptions of self of a healthy person? How does this person manage the physical requirements of a sexual life with such an injury?

◆ Brown & Williams's (1995) research indicates women's feelings of self-worth are affected by the experience of arthritis. How might an increasingly arthritic hip affect the sexual life of a previously active independent person? Have you an example of this from discussion with a patient?

◆ What is your experience with the language of sexuality? Do you find it comes easily to you? Have you an experience of developing an understanding of acceptable sexual words when working with a patient in your own practice?

What do you think are the responsibilities of the practitioner when exploring the losses in these examples? When working alone, relate your ideas to your own practice.

Reflection point 5.3

Working in a group, take the opportunity to discuss the common difficulties experienced when discussing feelings with a patient and whether it seemed to help. Did the patient say it was helpful? Did you ask the patient; if not, why not? Would you consider this question to be part of your evaluation of practice?

Discussion of the language of sexuality could be helpful in comparing different ways colleagues find of doing this. What are the different difficulties that members of the group have found when discussing sexuality with patients? Is it usually easier for men to discuss sexuality with men, and women with women? What are the implications for developing practice?

The pain of mental illness

There is a chilling story by Kafka (1992) describing the increasing isolation of someone changed into an insect overnight and the subsequent isolation from, and rejection by, family and friends – a telling fable for the agony of transformation caused by the mental illness of a loved family member.

Specialist practitioners in mental health recognise how long-term mental illness can continue to damage relationships of all kinds. They work with the isolated person and the suffering caused in the patient, their family and other relationships. Mental health problems can damage and change relationships and the difficulties may be increased by the anxieties provoked in the community (see Chapter 12).

In the case study below, a simple question, asked with some diffidence, changed the relationship between Miss Indra and the volunteer from one of silent dependency to one of mutuality. An ordinary approach enabled a bridge to be built between two people.

Case study 5.3

Miss Indra was experienced by others as a taciturn lady, silent and withdrawn. She sometimes received a lift from a volunteer to allow her to attend a luncheon club at the weekends. She was previously a teacher but had been severely ill with schizophrenia for many years. She had made a partial recovery and now lived independently, supported by her GP and social worker. One day during a tense and silent drive the volunteer, wishing to deal with the difficult silence and open a conversation, asked, 'Do you think your illness has changed you?' Miss Indra responded with a surprising warmth and delight, 'Oh, you would not have known me before, I was so happy. I loved my job and working with children, I was a really nice person to know, I wish you could have known me then.'

Reflection point 5.4

It is not always easy to appreciate that mental illness can stimulate feelings of loss and grief. At the very least the individual, family and friends have lost the person they knew.

◆ What is your experience of the difference made to the practitioner–patient relationship when you show the patient you are interested in how they feel and how their life has been affected by their illness?

◆ What experience of psychiatric illness have you had in your practice? Was it possible to discuss their loss of mental health with the person concerned and how did you do so? What was the outcome?

Caring for the distress of loss

Feelings require acknowledgement not reassurance

Some practitioners have expressed the anxiety that when a patient does not mention their feelings about a troubling experience, then for the practitioner to do so is tantamount to putting words in the patient's mouth. They fear alerting the patient to some feelings of which they may have been previously unaware. The notion has also been expressed that if the worker raises the issue of feelings, unnecessary pain may be caused. Bea's story is an example where the contrary is true.

Bea's story is a description of a misunderstanding. The practitioner was alarmed by Bea's mention of her lonely crying and seemed to feel some responsibility to keep Bea happy and content. To do so, and to save precious time, she saw her task was to 'stem the flood' and not cause distress by accepting the story of tears or by making further enquiries, whereas the old lady's wish was to talk about her son. Apparently confused, Bea understood, however, the way her feelings were being side-lined and indicated this by her wink to her friend.

Case study 5.4

Bea is in her mid-80s. Now registered blind and suffering from multiple cerebral infarcts she is a lively woman who lives independently thanks to her team of home care assistants and friends. She came to the UK from central Europe as a young woman in the 1930s and has lived a very full life. In later life she nursed her husband at home until his death; her youngest son took his own life after this and along with these sadnesses her sight continued to degenerate as the macular degeneration became severe. She is also troubled by her increasing loss of memory, which embarrasses her. She easily becomes confused and the difference between dreaming and daily life is sometimes difficult for her to grasp.

One evening a practitioner visiting her at home when a friend was there, remarked that Bea had a broken blood vessel in her left eye. Bea said that it did not trouble her; she offered the explanation that she had been crying a lot. The practitioner jollied her along saying that she had seemed very happy over the weekend and had not seemed at all sad. Bea said, 'Ah, but you don't know how I am when I'm alone here,' and looked across to her friend and winked. Later, alone with the friend, Bea remarked she was missing her son a lot at the moment and had been feeling especially sad and lonely. They were able to talk together about memories of him and Bea remarked that she liked to talk about him even though it made her sad.

Reassurance is for the reassurer

John Diamond (1998) describing his experiences as a cancer sufferer writes:

> *I'd come to the conclusion that whenever somebody told me how much good a positive attitude would do me, what they meant was how much easier a positive attitude would make it for them. Positivism meant we could all carry on as before ... As long as I was positive it meant they did not have to cope with nasty thoughts.*

The pain of listening to feelings of distress

Reassurance might be understood as another way of saying 'be quiet, please do not trouble me, I do not wish to share in your pain' – a hard way of looking at a response that tends to be offered when the practitioner might be feeling lost and helpless in a situation. However, the recognition of such feelings is an asset to understanding how the patient is feeling. Could it be that they both share similar feelings of being lost and helpless? It is when the practitioner is brave enough to stop, think about the feelings and see the link with the patient, that proper attention can be paid to the pain.

We might ask, on such occasions, whose pain is being considered, patient or practitioner? The recipient's perception of reassurance is not one of comfort; it is seen as minimising the authenticity of their distress. Listening and talking with people about their painful feelings can be troubling and painful for the practitioner. When this is faced squarely and seen as part of the process of care, then the patient has an opportunity to make an alliance, which means that they are no longer alone with their distress (see Chapter 6).

Recapitulation

Loss damages the sense of self, which in turn leads to changes in the concept of the sexual self. Skills of listening and understanding can support the process of change and help to integrate the experience of loss

Loss → Disturbance to sense of self → Change in concept of sexual self

When a patient's painful feelings are discussed and recognised as belonging to the patient then the practitioner does not carry them away. The feelings remain with the patient until integrated into the personality, which takes time. The effect of grief is different for each person. It is important that, however distressing recognising another's pain may be, the practitioner can help the patient keep the ownership of the feelings and move towards replanning their lives in a way that values the past.

The practitioner has the right to choose not to listen. There is no immunity to grief for any person and Parkes & Markus (1998) suggest that 'We need to find ways of distancing ourselves from the problems as well as tackling them.'

> **Reflection point 5.5**
>
> Examples in earlier chapters may be reconsidered in the light of this discussion on loss (for example Mr James, Chapter 2, pp 25–26). Consider, too, the losses and depression experienced by a stoma patient.
>
> ◆ How might loss affect the sexual feelings of patients in your practice?
>
> ◆ Do you have ideas about any developments in your own practice which could allow for recognition of and work with these issues?
>
> ◆ Have you written about any feelings you experience when working with loss and sexuality in your reflective diary?

Considerations of the effect of some losses met by patients

Grief is the normal reaction to loss and is the means by which people begin to accept the reality of an event which will change their lives. (Parkes & Markus 1998, p. 11)

Having considered impairment to health as a major contributor to feelings of loss and distress we can now study some specific examples of loss experienced in everyday clinical care and the potential effect that grief about this loss has upon sexual health.

Preparation for loss is of the utmost importance. When it is clear to clinicians that loss of whatever kind is inevitable, there is a responsibility to prepare the patient. Clear information given at the patient's pace, and opportunities to explore and be supported through the feelings that arise, can make a difference to managing the suffering of grief, pain and loss. The practitioner's role in preparing for loss is discussed again at the end of this chapter.

Continence

The problems associated with elimination are particularly sensitive because they also interfere with the sense of self. Along with this disturbance to both normality and the desire for cleanliness, clients may have to cope with appliances which also disturb their body image and may produce a sense of shame. Their normal feelings of attractiveness are disarrayed. Help may be required to retain a sense of self – including a sexual self. The patient may feel unclean and withdraw from relationships because they are unable to imagine that others can find them attractive.

Some drug treatments contributing to loss of sexual function

Practitioners are sometimes asked for help about loss of orgasm or libido following surgery, radiotherapy or other medical treatments.

In a recent article, Gamlin (1999) issues a challenge to practitioners to recognise that concerns about sexuality and body image remain unaddressed despite considerable literature on the subject. He suggests that neither the physiological component nor the effect of various drugs especially when taken on a long-term basis should be overlooked. Some drugs may contribute to sexual dysfunction. He gives a list which is useful as a reference to aid practitioners:

◆ Tobacco and alcohol
◆ Beta-adrenoreceptor blocking drugs – propanol
◆ Diuretics – bendrofluazide and spironolactone
◆ Hormones – goserelin and buserelin
◆ H2 receptor antagonists – cimetidine
◆ Proton pump inhibitors – omeprazole
◆ Antihypertensives – clonidine, methyldopa and captopril
◆ Lipid-lowering drugs – bezafibrate
◆ Anxiolytics – diazepam
◆ Antipsychotics – chlorpromazine and flupenthixol
◆ Antidepressants – amitryptyline and some serotonin re-uptake inhibitors
◆ Anti-epileptics – carbamazepine.

Some other causes for dysfunction

Illnesses such as advancing diabetes can seriously impair sexual function, causing loss of erection in both sexes. Radiotherapy for cancer of the pelvic region may give rise to shrinking and hypertrophy of organs. Following pelvic irradiation it is important for the vagina to remain patent. Once healing has occurred, patients are encouraged to regularly stretch the vagina by using fingers or dilators. The resumption of full penetrative intercourse also helps. For some people this handling of their vagina is too difficult. Whether research will show that these particular women have always been shy of taking an interest in their vagina and previously had difficulty touching and owning their genitalia, we do not know. Perhaps their experience of treatment has been to hand over their body to another and they feel that they have no right to 'own' it again. The result, however, is that the untouched irradiated vagina is in danger of hypertrophy, becoming hard and impenetrable even to the examining finger for follow-up treatment. Questions remain of how to understand and help in this situation where the vagina has become 'lost' to the woman.

Some surgical procedures – radical hysterectomy and prostatectomy or radical surgery to the gut – cause damage to nerve pathways, leading to partial or complete loss of sexual function. When the operation is performed as a life-saving measure, for example following pelvic cancer in men or women, it may lead to complete loss of sensation, which can be shattering to the shared life of a couple.

Everett (1998), writing of the effects of vasectomy says, 'some men experience signs of grief over their loss of fertility and sexuality. This will depend on how the man feels about his decision; if he feels forced or coerced into the decision then he may feel anger and sadness over his loss.'

Practitioner awareness of some effects of lowered libido

When libido is lowered a number of things happen. The patient will become aware of the loss of their usual sexual drive, as does their partner. Sensitivity to the likelihood of some partner misunderstandings is important and the practitioner's alertness to verbal or gestural clues to this difficulty is vital in the care of the couple. For some, a partner's loss of libido can only mean that they are involved with another person.

Greer (1999) writes, 'A woman is likely to interpret lack of erection in her male partner as evidence of lack of desire and hence lack of affection. Because she associates desire with affection, she believes that her partner must too.'

A woman experiencing loss of libido is unlikely to mention this; she is more likely to blame herself than see the links with prescribed drugs, other treatments or radical surgery. Therefore she is unlikely to recognise the possibility of help and it is even more important for the practitioner to be prepared to raise the issue. The loss of satisfaction can even be missed by the partner, when orgasms may be 'faked' to keep the experience from being felt as a failure by that loved person.

The loss of never having had

Practitioners occasionally encounter the loss of 'never having had' and 'never going to have now'. Necessary gynaecological operations which destroy the chance of having a baby, a hysterectomy for example, can rouse feelings of loss in some, even when the operation is likely to be life-saving. For some it can be experienced as the end of their future as a sexual woman whilst others may feel free of what had come to be felt as a burden.

Testicular cancer in a man may also be experienced in this way, especially if the lump was noticed but was ignored and sterility results. The sense of self-blame may damage the ability to really mourn those losses, especially when childlessness results.

A life-threatening tubal pregnancy not only means the loss of the pregnancy but may threaten future fertility. The work of grief here is likely to be complex and, when not addressed, may have implications for future sexual life.

Facing infertility is an occasion for mourning and grief and requires trained and sensitive support. Feelings can swing between hope and despair and people can be left with a complex set of emotions such as increasing irritability, resentment and loss of sexual libido, which are all symptoms of grief. The sense of blame between some partners is particularly distressing for practitioners who have been involved with the couple. Skilled counselling is required and both the patient and the counsellor can be supported by the sensitivity of other staff in the unit.

Many questions arise about the effect upon feelings, sexual activity and sexual life following these experiences. It may take many counselling sessions for a couple to be able to hold their feelings of anger and grief mutually (see Chapter 11).

Another never-having-had loss is a source of shame and secrecy (H Lowther, unpublished work, 1997) and seems unlike other difficulties met with in this area of the body. Practitioners who work in gynaecology, family planning and infertility services meet some women who have never been able to achieve penetrative intercourse. For some of these women touching, using tampons

---

Reflection point 5.6

It is impossible to overstress that preparation for loss is vital. Read this poem and reflect upon its possible effect on your practice.

This woman's body

There is so much this woman's body of mine has never known
the abuse of violation
the degradation of poverty
the despoilation of conquest or invasion
the mutilation of war and pillage and rape
and the weight of a baby in her belly
and the spilling of a body from between her legs
the pull of a mouth on milk-filled breasts
the tug of a life on her overflowing heart
the long tangled years of mothering, cherishing, separating,
never separating and the comfort of growing old with a mate
And for all these curses and blessings
which she will never know
I hold and honour her now.

Nicola Slee (unpublished work, 1997) with permission

or even imagining the vagina and vulval area cause feelings of disgust and distress. This is not a question of intellectual knowledge of anatomy but is about troubled and hidden feelings. It seems for most of these women as though their vagina does not belong to them. Each woman seeking help requires trained and experienced psychosexual counselling if she desires to take ownership of this area of her body. One woman after treatment said, 'I never thought we would do it. It was so easy. All those years of pain and it was nothing really extraordinary.'

For the practitioner, once again the need is to discover meanings for each individual person.

The individual response

In a group discussion with oncology specialist practitioners, there was a suggestion that for some women, a hysterectomy is experienced as loss of womanhood and femininity (see Chapter 12). One practitioner found this idea difficult, and gave an alternative example of a patient whom she had known and treated with radiotherapy for some time, described below.

The discussion again highlighted the need to understand each individual as having specific needs and feelings. There are no short cuts to knowing people. Understanding and recognition of the person's response to their illness or disease is paramount in the helping environment.

The continuing care for loss and grief in aiding recovery

People do emerge through grief to live full and active lives again and return to their sense of themselves as whole and sexual beings. Practitioners' help is valuable in supporting this emergence.

Skrine (1997) writes, 'the reaction of grief and loss is an intensely personal one, and each of us has to negotiate mourning of our losses in his or her own way.'

Case study 5.5

The young and lively patient with two small children had received lengthy radiotherapy treatment. As a result of her illness she had experienced and coped with a wide variety of surgical treatment involving a mastectomy, a hysterectomy, oophorectomy, a nephrectomy and lost her hair. She had coped with all this and lived a full life with partner and children. Now there is a threat of requiring more surgery which would result in a stoma. For her, this is the threat to her femininity and so far she feels unable to cope with it.

Feelings take time to emerge. When the patient has had opportunity to recover from the initial physical shock of illness or surgery and recovery is beginning, awareness of the whole experience will begin. This is a time of sensitivity and the practitioner's skills are tested. The task is to be alert to the time that the person is ready and wishes to talk over feelings about their experience of the event.

Within modern health practice, patients spend only a short time in hospital following the interventions of medicine and surgery. The 'complication' is that there is often no time to begin the work of supporting feelings in the acute setting. It is when the feelings remain inside, unexplored and unintegrated into the personality, that other practitioners are likely to meet unexplained reactions from patients in different settings. In general practice, unexplained physical disturbances may be related to such issues. Health visitors, for example, can find opportunities to follow-up after stillbirth when the mother returns home quickly from hospital.

Unexplored, painful feelings do not go away. An example is Robert's story in Chapter 3 (pp 55–56). There the distress about sexuality exposed in the well man clinic was the complication of a life lived full of unintegrated and confused feelings about the self. These were brought about by brief surgery in childhood with no opportunity to understand until years later.

Helping to bring about some resolution of grieving

It is important to recognise that many people say they have not got over their sadness. Sadness often stays with a person following loss, like 'a bruise on the heart' (Morley 1992), which may distress friends and family who feel that the work of grief should mean that the loss and sadness are no longer talked about (see Chapter 10). However that is not always the case – see Bea's story earlier in this chapter.

Some resolution of grieving is, however, usually achieved in a way that makes possible the continuation of living, the scars remaining to the end of life. Walter (1996) writes of 'enabling the living to integrate the memory of the dead into their ongoing lives.' The indication of resolution beginning is a sense of new reality; a different and whole self can be experienced with the integration of the lost part.

A practitioner speaks of helping a young couple complete some of their work of grief in the following case study (E Bordass, unpublished work, 1999).

Case study 5.6

Some hospital chaplaincies and other places of worship advertise ceremonies where grieving people are able to spend shared quiet time in contemplation of their loss with a few readings and some music. Losses may be different, perhaps a still-born child, a miscarriage, a termination of pregnancy, a diagnosis

Case study 5.6 (cont'd)

of severe illness, the discovery that a couple have been found to be infertile, a relationship ending. All, however, are causes for grief; all are 'might-have-beens'.

A young woman came for contraceptive advice. The nurse noticed that she had undergone a termination of pregnancy in the previous few months and asked how she was. She told the story of how she and her boyfriend, very much in love, had been shocked to find her pregnant. They considered their personal situation was impossible to maintain a pregnancy. Supported by friends and family they had decided to terminate the pregnancy. It had seemed the only course of action at the time.

Now they found themselves still grieving for the baby that might have been. The family and friends had been a great support, but the couple just could not let the guilt and sadness go.

The nurse suggested to them that some people found a ceremony helpful in completing a period of sadness and loss. They discussed the possibilities together. The girl had an idea of floating a cork with a lighted candle to sail away down the river in a ceremony shared with close friends, which might enable them to 'let go'.

Gay and lesbian people sometimes find funerals and bereavement a time of special difficulty, especially when their love for the dead person was hidden and they had not 'come out' to relatives and friends. There is special need for recognition and help when feeling isolated with grief. The Gay and Lesbian Bereavement Project is available to help. The office is staffed from Monday to Thursday (Tel: 0208 200 0511) and a member is on duty in the evenings (Tel: 0208 455 8894).

For many life-changing events there is no recognised religious ceremony or ritual to help with the work of grief. Some people have found it helpful to make their own ceremony, perhaps planting a tree or building a cairn, writing some words of farewell or setting aside a quiet time to share memories with close friends and family. The opportunity to mark the moving on from grieving may help. The memory of the loss remains as a part of the person.

A lady of 79 spoke of the loss of her fourth child from diphtheria aged 3, 54 years before. She described her memories of the chubby arms supporting the chin and the smiling baby-face as she had sat at the family table all those years ago. She had never forgotten her and shed a tear as she remembered. In her document box she still had the black-edged death notice. She had lived a full life, had two more children and now had numerous much loved grandchildren, but she still remembered Gladys with love.

Reflection point 5.7

Take a moment or two to consider this piece of writing. Listen to the words and listen to the 'music', that inner meaning which the words convey.

> The bodies of grownups
> come with stretchmarks and scars,
> faces that have been lived in,
> relaxed breasts and bellies,
> backs that give trouble,
> and well worn feet:
> flesh that is particular
> and obviously mortal.
> They also come
> with bruises on their heart,
> wounds they can't forget, and each of them
> a company of lovers in their soul
> who will not return
> and cannot be erased.
> And yet I think there is a flood of beauty
> beyond the smoothness of youth;
> and my heart aches for that grace of longing
> that flows through bodies
> no longer straining to be innocent,
> but yearning for redemption.

(Janet Morley 1992, with permission)

◆ Does this poem help you to be aware of feelings sometimes alerted in you by physical care? Consider what the words mean for you in terms of your own practice. Do they make you think of someone in particular? Are you reminded of a particular occasion or event in your clinical work? You might care to reflect upon that memory and its meaning for you and why you have remembered it.

◆ Some patients seem to teach us a great deal about care. Is there one patient in particular that you learned something from that affected or improved your practice?

◆ Is there anything that you recognise in this poem that has implications for your own practice in caring for sexuality?

◆ Do you know of any arrangements locally for ceremonies relating to ending a period of grief? How do you see your role in helping to complete the work of grief with patients and families in your practice?

Working in a group: When working on this together, listen to one person reading carefully and slowly and leave space for thought before considering and discussing the implications it may have for individuals when considering the issues above.

Reflections on understandings gained from care

Bodies, along with words, minds and feelings (including those about sexuality) are the focus for the work of the health care professional. Poetry seems to have more impact and becomes more accessible when read out loud. So, read out loud the poem in Reflection point 5.7. Take time to listen as you read it slowly for yourself.

The practitioner's role in preparing patients for likely effects of treatment

Some losses happen suddenly, death or accident for example; however, with most medical and surgical procedures there is time to prepare the patient. Once again it is important to understand that preparation for a loss to the self can help with the feelings that may follow.

The proper preparation for treating an illness, prior to surgery or the use of a particular drug, is discussing with the patient any likelihood of effects on themselves or their sexual function. This is usually the responsibility of the doctor member of the team. Other members of the team will need to know what the patient has been told so that sexual health care may be in accord during recovery.

Preparation can help in the process of dealing with the losses that are to come. When preparation is neglected, the patient will soon become aware of the change but may not understand the role of treatment. This in turn may lead to self-blame and loss of self-worth. When the tasks of preparation and explanation are avoided by health care practitioners, the human misery involved cannot be overstated.

CONCLUSION

It is interesting to notice how often news of a death can provoke stories and memories of other deaths. All have experiences of loss and memories can be reawakened on hearing news of any death. Practitioners are not immune to sad feelings when witnessing death. This can be especially difficult when it is a patient known and cared for. It can be painful to feel helpless in the face of death and grief. It remains important to recognise and accept feelings of grief and sadness in ourselves if we are to remain alert to them in others.

Painful feelings are worthy of care, and opportunities should be sought to speak about them in a supportive setting. Unexplored painful feelings do not go away (see Chapter 6, Taking care of the practitioner).

Caring for sexuality includes recognising and understanding how the experience of loss can often change the image of the self. It may be easier to understand the grief that follows death than the distress felt at some other losses, which can be intense, hidden by shame and hard to recognise. The practitioner's listening skills and her offer to explore and understand such feelings of loss can make a difference to how a patient recovers.

BIBLIOGRAPHY

Parkes C M, Markus A 1998 Coping with loss: helping patients and their families. BMJ Publications, London
This book covers a variety of losses likely to occur during the lifespan and demonstrates that the right help at the right time can reduce psychological harm caused by major losses.

Pincus L 1997 Death in the family. Faber and Faber, London
Practitioners will find useful insights into the continuing effects of grief and concepts to help in their responses in practice.

Agencies that can be contacted for help include the following:

Cruse Bereavement Care. Telephone 0181 940 4818

Compassionate Friends. Telephone 0117 953 9639

Diamond J 1998 C: because cowards get cancer too ... Vermillion, London
This book, written by a journalist, gives a not-always-comfortable patient's-eye view of the cancer services and treatment he experienced.

Cort E 1998 Nurses' attitudes to sexuality in caring for cancer patients. Nursing Times 94 (42): 54–56
This presents a challenging and helpful survey of nurses' attitudes to terminally ill cancer patients.

Lewis C S 1961 A grief observed. Faber & Faber, London
A personal and moving account of grief. Also adapted to stage and screen as 'Shadowlands'.

Mathieson C M, Stamm H J 1995 Renegotiating identity: cancer narratives. Society of Health and Illness 17(3): 283–306
This research paper illustrates through case examples how cancer creates new experiences and a new identity, but this is not a passive experience: identities are renegotiated.

REFERENCES

Brown S, Williams A 1995 Womens' experiences of rheumatoid arthritis. Journal of Advanced Nursing 21: 695–701

Cookson C 1999 On the alert for cries of pain. Financial Times (13/14 February)

Diamond J 1998 C: because cowards get cancer too. Vermillion, London

Everett S 1998 Handbook of contraception and family planning. Baillière Tindall, London, Ch 3, p 59

Gamlin R 1999 Sexuality: a challenge for nursing practice. Nursing Times 95(7): 48–50

Greer G 1999 ... or a soft option. The Observer (24 January)

Kafka F 1992 The complete short stories: The Metamorphosis. Minerva, London

Kaplan S, Greenfield S, Ware J 1989 Assessing the effects of physician–patient interactions on the outcomes of chronic disease. Medical Care 27(3) (suppl): 110–127

Macklin D, Heslop A, Rosser R 1983 Breathlessness and psychiatric morbidity in chronic bronchitis and emphysema: a study of psychotherapeutic management. Psychological Medicine 13: 93–110

Mathieson C M, Stamm H J 1995 Renegotiating identity: cancer narratives. Society of Health and Illness 17(3): 283–306

Morley J 1992 The bodies of grownups. All desires known. SPCK, London

Murray F 1999 Don't mention the, er. Guardian (21 January)

Parkes C M, Markus A 1998 Coping with loss. BMJ Publications, London, Ch 1, pp 2, 6, 7, 11

Pincus L 1997 Death in the family. Faber & Faber, London, Ch 6, pp 112–129; Ch 7, p 131

Skrine R 1997 Blocks and freedoms in sexual life. Radcliffe Medical Press, Oxford, Ch 9, p 102

Steinem G 1998 Foreword. In: Ensler E The Vagina Monologues. Villard Books, New York

Walter T 1996 A new model of grief: bereavement and biography. Mortality 1(1):

6

Maintaining and developing professional skills and taking care of the practitioner

Doreen Clifford

KEY ISSUES

◆ Balancing closeness and distance
◆ Reassurance is different from support
◆ The ability to hold projected feelings as part of care
◆ Understanding the link between patient's and practitioner's needs
◆ Resources for taking care of the practitioner

INTRODUCTION

This chapter is in two parts. The first looks at some of the ways in which the delicate balance of closeness and distance between patient and practitioner may be understood, maintained and managed. The second continues the theme of how practitioners themselves require care when maintaining a therapeutic potential in the patient–practitioner relationship and reviews resources available to help.

THE MAINTENANCE OF A BALANCE IN CARE

Like a tightrope walker along a high wire, one of the most fascinating and difficult things to manage is a professional balance in care. As skills develop, understanding grows of the need to maintain a sense of oneself as separate but involved and as distinct but not distant from patients and clients. When balance is lost there is danger of falling into one of two difficult ways of working:

◆ over-involvement
◆ non-involvement.

Maintaining the balance between closeness and distance

Preserving the sense of each person, patient and practitioner as distinct individuals is beset with many difficulties. Over-involvement can interfere with appropriate care, damage the professional self and the working relationship between practitioner and patient. On such occasions confusions arise, making it difficult to distinguish between professional relationships and friendship. Of course this does not mean that professional caring relationships should not be friendly and co-equal partnerships. Nevertheless, it is important to distinguish between the professional relationship and friendship.

Donald Winnicott is quoted as saying that 'Friendliness of approach and sincerity of care tenders a space between client and practitioner. Within this space, the patient has opportunity to make clear their needs and preoccupations and the professional has opportunity to listen and respond. Personalisation of one's own feelings denies the patient's requirement for space to be an individual and the resulting confusion obscures their needs for respect and help'.

When the pain expressed by the patient is intense then it may be difficult to maintain the professional self. A patient may show pain through anger, sadness, depression or a lack of self-worth. Being close to intense feelings can draw the practitioner towards the patient. If, however, the practitioner crosses the boundary and moves into the patient's space then the therapeutic opportunity may be lost.

Case study 6.1

Angela Green came to a clinic to get advice about contraception. Whilst discussing options with the practitioner she became distressed and tearful. The practitioner wondered how she could help as Angela, tears flowing, told her that suddenly becoming aware of the date had reminded her that this was the anniversary of the loss of a much wanted baby late in pregnancy. Touched and saddened at the story, the practitioner began to reassure Angela, going on to say that she understood the pain of this, having herself experienced such a loss. She said that she too still shed tears on occasion. The patient stopped crying; instead she expressed her sorrow and understanding for the practitioner.

Several different things occurred in Angela's story:

◆ The patient became distressed, when reminded by the date.
◆ The practitioner showed concern and learned about the loss of the baby.
◆ The practitioner was touched by the story and the pain alerted a memory of her own.
◆ She used her own painful memory as an attempt to reassure the patient.

The patient did not receive help for her pain, instead she stopped crying and turned her attention to the practitioner who seemed to be in need.

The lost opportunities were:

◆ The patient was prevented from talking over her sadness with a professional.
◆ The patient's sadness was not recognised as appropriate (Nichols 1993) to the sad memory of her loss of a baby.
◆ There was no opportunity to discuss whether this sadness was affecting her life, her relationships or her love-making.
◆ The practitioner was unable to use her psychosexual skills to help this woman.

Angela's story seems to suggest that the practitioner may need a place to consider what the experience of her own loss of a baby meant. Without this reflection it seems likely that the practitioner's own feelings may be alerted and impel her into the patient's therapeutic space again.

The practitioner felt she wanted to comfort the patient and so said that she understood the pain. A practitioner's hope of giving 'reassurance' through telling her own story, being positive (as in Chapter 5), or other interventions which distract from the patient's pain are commonplace, but leave the patient isolated. Quoting her tutor, Fabricius (1991) has described reassurance as 'like isolating a fire in a fire blanket – it stopped you catching alight but left the patient burning alone.'

When practitioners are supported by colleagues they are less likely to turn away from a patient's pain. The practitioner who recognises the patient's pain may, in a sense, 'hold' some of that pain for the patient (Menzies 1960, Fabricius 1991, de Lambert 1997). This in itself is often therapeutic. The activity of getting someone else involved in one's own pain is often so forceful, it is as though the pain is being thrown into another person. Babies and young children survive and develop through having some of their pain 'held' by parents and carers. For most people, physical and psychological distress stimulates a similar need – for someone else to hold and share the pain. This is probably a major contribution to recovery, albeit often unacknowledged. It has been described as 'projection'. 'Reassurance', Fabricius suggests, 'is a way of refusing to accept a patient's projections.' Menzies (1960) draws attention to the force of projection in health care: 'Patients and relatives treat the staff in such a way as to ensure that the (nurses) experience these feelings instead of – or partly instead of – themselves.'

The differences between support and reassurance

When working in a situation where the professional self is under strain, support from other people is helpful and can aid the maintenance of confidence in one's ability to tackle the task. The feeling of being supported seems to arise from the experience of being understood. Easy judgements are set aside and we feel at one with the person offering us support, e.g. when a colleague recognises that a situation is difficult and offers neither criticism nor advice, but lets us know that they recognise that we are coping with an uncomfortable situation.

How does support come about? It seems best when the people concerned see themselves as co-equal in the situation. Their shared professionalism allows the support to happen. Neither profession nor experience are allowed to get in the way of two adults who somehow recognise the need of the other through either a glance or an offer of words. Most of us have experienced shared professionalism and often a bond is forged which supports the work. What we learn from such occasions can help in the development of our own skills for supporting patients. Once again, the feeling of support comes from being understood.

Reflection point 6.1

◆ In your practice are you aware of the variety of roles you occupy for different people as changes in treatment progress?

◆ How would you compare the role you need to play with a physically ill, dependent person to that you need to play with one recovering well?

◆ Do you have an awareness of 'holding' feelings for a patient at times of illness and other times of difficulty?

◆ Can you remember a time when you accepted and 'held' feelings of pain for a patient? What did that feel like and what was the outcome?

◆ Do you remember a time when that was too difficult and you found yourself reassuring them rather than 'getting involved'? Do you remember the feelings you had then?

◆ What does the description of the 'fire-blanket' of reassurance mean in your own practice?

Looking back through previous chapters you can see this concept of projection of feelings in some of the stories told. What difference might this understanding make to your own practice?

Working in a group could be valuable. If you are brave enough to describe and compare occasions when you retreated into reassurance with a patient, you may grow a clearer picture of how this seems to come about. You may also think of ways in which it could be possible to develop the 'holding' skill of the practitioner, the support you would then need and how you could develop this support within the group.

Staying away from the patient or offering a bridge?

Keeping oneself aloof from involvement does not avoid the difficulty. Most people are aware of the experience of feeling ignored when seeking a service. We quickly become alert to places such as shops and offices where the service personnel are more interested in a personal conversation than in paying attention to customers. This experience can be mirrored when seeking advice from a professional who does not make eye contact but focuses on a writing pad or computer screen rather than paying attention to us. On such occasions we are left feeling neglected, impatient and extremely irritated and will probably decide to try elsewhere another time.

Jeremy Hardy (1997) articulated something of this experience:

> *But it seems to happen in many professions that the training loses sight of the fact that the jobs involve interaction with human beings. This results in the rudeness of Post Office counter staff, the insensitivity of consultant physicians, the patronising superiority of social workers and the tendency among police officers to want to get as much of the population as possible into prison with the greatest possible haste.*

You may find this an overstatement, but the sense of non-involvement as a damaging experience is clearly expressed here.

In retreat from a relationship

Non-involvement can arise for many reasons, as when the practitioner is not in touch with the whole of herself and her defences are aroused, perhaps by personal pain, tiredness, stress or private preoccupations. Sometimes it is the client who seemingly rejects the offer of an opportunity to use the professional relationship. It may be that their inner turmoil is such that the projection system they inhabit is one surrounded by adversaries. The practitioner can join the ranks of these adversaries if not alert to the need to pay special attention to making a more useful relationship.

The following is an example of a practitioner who was able to respond to a woman demonstrating alienating behaviour almost as though she was not seeking help.

Case study 6.2

It was a busy clinic and the practitioner needed material from the waiting area. She politely asked a patient to move to let her get at the cupboard. The patient was irritated, sighing and tutting, despite the rather ordinary situation. The practitioner was dismayed when later the same patient, frowning and grim-faced, came into her cubicle for attention. She was alerted to a potentially difficult situation by this woman's behaviour. Rather than challenge the irritated woman, she said, 'You look as though you would rather not be here today.' The patient gave her a long look and started to weep. She went on to share her feelings of anger and despair at the relationship with her partner and her fears for their future.

The skilful practitioner recognised that something difficult was likely to occur in the practitioner–patient relationship, which allowed her to pay attention to the patient's feelings. The practitioner recognised that the disquiet she felt about this apparently 'difficult' woman belonged to the patient and offered a neutral observation about her perception of the woman not wanting to be at the clinic. The observation was accepted, allowing the patient to trust the practitioner with the distress she was carrying. We might describe this as not accepting the patient's projection of the practitioner as an adversary.

Reflection point 6.2

The story above may be familiar to you and may remind you of strategies you have used on similar occasions in your own practice. You may find it useful to reflect upon and write about two contrasting occasions:

◆ Describe an occasion when you felt able to resist the projection to be a particular kind of practitioner and were able to remain yourself (as in the story above).

◆ Can you recall another time when you were not so successful and behaved perhaps in a cross, insincere or conciliatory way, which in retrospect seems inappropriate?

Working in a group: in discussion with colleagues, can you discover ways of supporting each other to study such events as interesting and important, to develop further skills?

> **Reflection points for the coach 6.3**
>
> Anxiety about involvement diminishes care not only for the practitioner but also for learners and others supervised by the practitioner (Menzies 1960).
>
> ◆ Have you read Menzies' original paper recently? Reading and comparing the institution described by her and that in which you work could be challenging.
>
> ◆ What defences against anxiety exist in the social system in which you practice?
>
> ◆ What steps do you and your colleagues take to amend this to improve the care of students, colleagues and therefore patients?

Continuing care

Intimacy in the practitioner–patient relationship

As confidence in sexual health care grows and skills increase there are times when, because one has dared to listen, tender and intimate events and memories may be spoken about. The practitioner who has dared to listen may become the valued recipient of the patient's thoughts and feelings which have been brought to mind by the circumstances of illness or treatment. This intimacy can touch deep feelings of the practitioner's own experience and on many occasions can deepen the bond already existing between practitioner and patient.

Where sharing understandings and the development of psychosocial skills is seen as a focus, then tenderness in the practitioner–patient relationship is recognised as part of the caring environment, which holds possibilities for healing (Savage 1995).

However, in other environments, such tenderness may be seen as questionable. It is important that the practitioner recognises when this is so and takes steps to safeguard their professional self from misunderstandings by colleagues, as in the case study below.

There are several important points to understand in this story:

◆ The willingness of the practitioner to accept the projection of sad and tender memories and to 'hold' them both physically and emotionally.
◆ Although aware of the likelihood of criticism by a colleague, the practitioner completed her work with the patient.
◆ The practitioner took care of the patient and herself by reporting his distress, and her response, to the manager.
◆ Observed by another, this way of working seemed not to be understood and provoked anxiety about the appropriateness of the practitioner's behaviour.

Case study 6.3

The practitioner was working in a nursing home and had the particular care of an elderly man who had spoken of how much he was missing his wife since her death in recent years. It was the practice in the establishment that for privacy the patient's room door was closed when attending to their care. One morning the practitioner noticed that the patient was sitting hunched in bed, his head low and obviously distressed. She put her arms around his shoulders and asked if she could help. He in turn put his arms around her too and wept. She comforted him and he said, 'I have not had my arms around a woman since my wife died.' The practitioner accepted this statement and was moved. At that moment another practitioner entered the room, gave a strained look and left quickly.

The elderly man's personal care was completed and the practitioner left the room. Alerted by the response of her colleague, she went to see the manager to report the man's distress and said that x had seen them in an embrace. The manager had already had this event reported to her but was pleased that the practitioner had come to tell her own story.

Taking care of one's self is complex. It is important to be aware of one's own needs, as the practitioner was in the last story, but it is difficult to develop psychosexual skills without the support of colleagues. When practitioners feel free to query, comment and voice their feelings, then skills can be examined and developed.

Reflection point 6.4

Some teams of workers are able to maintain a mutually supportive working environment. In reflecting on your own professional life, no doubt you have mixed views and experiences of such events.

◆ What effect do you think the psychosocial environment has upon patient care?

◆ To feel safe to practise the care of sexuality, what kind of environment would you describe as likely to be supportive and encouraging?

◆ Do you have the authority to plan changes in your psychosocial system and to offer more support for skill development than at present?

◆ What help and support would you need to do this? Can you obtain this and from whom?

The link between patient needs and practitioner needs

The thinking so far about the continuing response to patient needs leads into the rest of this chapter, which is about the needs the practitioner has for gaining support and insight for developing skills.

TAKING CARE OF THE PRACTITIONER

Both attrition rates and sickness rates tend to rise when staffing numbers and/or skills are below the level required; morale falls and many practitioners feel unable to continue. There is a close link between the care of the practitioner and the standards of patient care. With continuing training, practitioners develop their confidence and their skills.

Time and energy spent on continuing training and support of practitioners is cost-effective for both practitioner and patient, and is the most effective method of support for developing confidence in practice. From confidence comes increased ability, the willingness to take risks and the advance of skill in patient care practice.

Resources for the professional needs of the practitioner

Reflective practice

Reflective practice is not an academic exercise but a living opportunity to develop skill using the study of one's own clinical work, alone, as part of a structured seminar training group (Clifford 1998), or in the informally structured groups described below (see Chapter 13). Benner's (1984) argument that skill is developed from the laying bare of knowledge embedded in practice, has been described in Chapter 4. Reflective practice has the great value of 'making skills visible' and therefore more freely available to the professional.

In previous chapters there has been a focus on the needs of the practitioner when difficult and painful memories and feelings are revealed by a patient. It may be useful to refresh your thinking on this subject by referring to reflective points 6.2, 6.3 and 6.4 and the notes for clinical managers in Chapter 4.

Keeping a reflective diary The uses of reflection on practice are manifold. A reflective diary can be a personal support in recognising and planning strategies to deal with common difficulties that are bound to arise (see Chapter 4).

In brief, it offers opportunity to:

◆ reflect upon clinical confidence and current skills
◆ recognise areas of difficulty, especially those encountered on more than one occasion

◆ reflect upon psychosexual pain described by a patient and take time to understand and consider one's responses
◆ consider and plan how to develop skills in responding to patients.

Group reflective practice Working with a group of colleagues engaged in similar work is often beneficial; when members share similar anxieties and difficulties the development of psychosexual skills is enhanced. Talking over clinical experiences and discussing the stories shared on these occasions can prove to be of great benefit in the development of understanding and expertise. Bowles (1995) argues that 'storytelling is an accessible yet powerful tool which contextualises and humanises (nursing) knowledge, facilitating a deeper understanding of self and others.'

The reflection points in this section could be used to help the group focus on specific issues. If you are having regular meetings you might like to choose two or three questions for each discussion.

Even if there are only two or three of you, set aside time to meet regularly. The support you gain from each other will be evident in the way your skills develop:

◆ in growing awareness of psychosexual issues
◆ recognising feelings in the practitioner
◆ understanding how often similar feelings are also present in the patient
◆ using this recognition to build bridges with patients to explore psychosexual and other distress
◆ developing the use of words to describe and explore feelings
◆ helping the move into involvement with patients to raise standards of care
◆ acknowledging skill development in each other.

Special interest groups In recent years some groups of practitioners have begun 'interest groups' in their specialty. For example in the north west of England there is a gynaeoncology interest group that meets every 2 months to share information, understandings and topics of professional interest.[1]

Psychosexual training seminars Section 3 of this book gives a detailed description of the use of Balint training seminars for the development of this work. We recommend that you seek out such training available in your geographical area.[2]

---

[1] For more information contact: The Macmillan Nurse, Liverpool Women's Hospital, Crown Street, Liverpool L8 7SS, UK
[2] For more information contact: The Association of Psychosexual Nursing, PO Box 2762, London W1A 5HQ, UK

Clinical supervision

Clinical supervision is another emerging method of support for practitioners.

In the past decade much has been written on the need for supervision in nursing but comparatively little has been written on effective techniques, or on the roles and requirements within the supervisory relationship.
(D Wells, unpublished work, 1998)

Butterworth & Faugier (1992) suggest 'that (practitioners) of all levels, from senior staff to students, require a relationship that focuses primarily on the process and experience of (care), is something the profession(s) have been slow to accept.' Rafferty (1998) says, 'My role as educational manager enables me to work with (practitioners) concerning what is supervision, and how it might be conducted. Such work has made it clear to me that supervision is something many (practitioners) long for.' Bulmer (1997) illustrates how supervision was implemented within a directorate in one Trust and that two-thirds of those receiving supervision valued it highly. He says, 'We believed clinical supervision would promote the development of primary nursing; support nurses exposed to changes in practice methods and care locations; and promote the role of F-grade nurses.'

Clinical supervision needs to fit the situation and the people, so there are few prescriptions, although Faugier puts forward some principles to guide a 'Growth and support model'. Balint seminar training fits Faugier's 'Growth and support model' (see Section 3). In the context of this chapter, the clinical supervisor is seen as someone who should be experienced in the specialty of the practitioner or in studying the skills used in that practice. The task is to help clarify difficulties, to expose the skills existing in practice and to support the development of the understandings and skills of daily practice.

Mentorship

For many practitioners, a mentor is an experienced colleague whose clinical expertise is trusted and who is met with regularly to discuss practice experiences, examples of clinical growth or difficulty and the development of skills in daily practice.

Training as a support system

The three areas of reflective practice, supervision and mentorship have in common the aim of supporting practice and practitioner. The Balint psychosexual seminar as a training and support system encompasses all three of these tasks (see Section 3).

In the context of this chapter, support is considered in three ways:

Recognition

> leading to

> > **Understanding**

> > leading to

> > > **Acknowledgement.**

Recognition of the individuality of the practitioner; their training, abilities, potentialities, developing skills, difficulties, strains and inevitable mistakes. **Understanding** of the situation of clinical care and the particular environment in which the practitioner works – whether this environment is supportive, critical or neutral. Relationships among the professional group of colleagues are explored and understood. Feelings provoked by patient care and in the practitioner–patient relationship are accepted. Discovering words to express feelings aroused by care and in the practitioner–patient relationship is assisted. **Acknowledgement** is given to the practitioner, the advances made in practice, difficulties experienced and plans for change.

The supportive relationship

Support exists within a relationship. Relationships with colleagues, a supervisor or a mentor all offer opportunities for support. Early in this chapter support was contrasted with reassurance: support usually takes place in a relationship that feels equal, whereas reassurance may leave the reassured feeling patronised.

So whose supportive relationship are we discussing here – practitioner's or patient's? It is clear that both the practitioner–patient relationship and the practitioner–supervisor/trainer relationship are closely allied. After all, the better the training and support of the practitioner, the better the standards of sensitive clinical care.

Seeking appropriate educational opportunities

Financial resources for continuing training exist within each division of health care and are usually managed by people who are ready to support training opportunities that are explained and make sense to them. It is important that practitioners understand their responsibility to seek out and use the education needed for their practice.

Becoming aware of the availability of workshops, study days, conferences and other opportunities related to psychosexual care is important. The networking at such events opens opportunities to understand that there are others struggling with this work and that there exists a variety of ways of working.

It is possible to arrange workshops, study days and seminar training for groups of people anywhere in the UK. Financial resources may sometimes be discovered from drug and dressing companies who may be willing to find money to support groups of practitioners.

Degree level studies in psychosexual care can be discovered by writing to local universities and colleges. For example, Greenwich University, London has a module in psychosexual awareness at levels two and three.

A summary of the arguments for continuing training systems

The link between continuing practitioner training and patient care is a close one. The opportunity to put feelings into words and explore those feelings with a trusted other offers the practitioner an experience of what may be achieved when feelings are recognised and understood. Such an experience is a paradigm and support for the practitioner–patient relationship.

In the absence of such an educational system, the practitioner's sensitivities are damaged, resulting in distancing as a strategy of defence. This is as true for a patient as for a practitioner; in the supported practitioner–patient relationship there are opportunities for both to find words for feelings. In similar discussions about feelings between patients and family and close friends, explorations can aid the sense of identity and the understandings needed during loss of health. The practitioner's experience of being recognised as an individual, understood and acknowledged, supports a standard of sensitive care that enhances the way in which patients, partners and relatives are cared for.

Personal and emotional health care needs of practitioners

Personal needs are the responsibility of the practitioner herself. It is important that when private pain levels are high, help is sought. Professional help of all kinds is available on the National Health Service and privately, and the GP is best placed to advise on gaining access to appropriate help. Counselling, psychotherapy, cognitive and behaviour therapies are all available, as are occupational health clinics offering advice and names and addresses of resources available. Personal grief, emotional pain and other difficulties should not be neglected.

Early in this chapter, a practitioner's story highlighted what may have been her unresolved grief. An occasion for personal counselling arises when private issues impinge upon clinical work, as in this example when the practitioner–patient relationship was interrupted by the worker's feelings aroused in the consultation. The recognition of the need for personal help is an important step towards recovery.

CONCLUSION

The work of holistic care, including recognition of the psychosexual elements in everyday practice, has been considered, argued and discussed in this section of the book.

Practitioners who previously have felt shy about integrating this aspect of work into their practice are encouraged to seek further training and to use colleagues to support them in the development of appropriate skills.

It is hoped that others who already recognise that many patients and clients welcome the opportunity to discuss intimate matters with them will have gained further ideas, confidence and support for their clinical work.

With the conclusion of this section of the book, the study of psychosexual care continues with interesting and stimulating reading about emotional development across the life span and training methods and opportunities.

BIBLIOGRAPHY

Johns C, Freshwater D 1998 Transforming nursing through reflective practice. Blackwell Science, Cambridge
A collection of papers from a 1997 conference on evaluating practice.

Parkes C M, Markus A 1998 Coping with loss. BMJ Books, London
Appendix A has a list of organisations providing training, advice or counselling to patients, their families and professional care givers.

Nichols K 1993 Psychological care in physical illness, 2nd edn. Chapman and Hall, London.
Chapter 7 offers many ideas for professional support and ways of making this useful to practitioners working with patients' feelings.

Workshops and study days can be arranged for groups of practitioners by The Association of Psychosexual Nursing. The Association holds two open study days a year in spring and autumn. For more information contact The Association of Psychosexual Nursing, PO Box 2762 London WIA 5HQ.

REFERENCES

Benner P 1984 From novice to expert: excellence and power in clinical nursing practice. Addison Wesley, Menlu Park, CA
Bowles N 1995 Storytelling: a search for meaning within nursing practice. Nurse Education Today 15: 365–369
Bulmer C 1997 Supervision: how it works. Nursing Times 93(48):
Butterworth T, Faugier J 1992 The supervisory relationship. In: Clinical supervision and mentorship in nursing. Stanley Thomas, London

Clifford D 1998 Psychosexual nursing seminars. In: Barnes E (ed) Face to face with distress. Butterworth Heinemann, London

de Lambert L 1998 Learning through experience. In: Barnes E (ed) Face to face with distress. Butterworth Heinemann, London

Fabricius J 1991 Running on the spot or can nursing really change? Psychoanalytic Psychotherapy 3(2): 97–108

Hardy J 1997 Evidence that was buried for decades. Guardian 1 Nov, 17

Johns C, Freshwater D 1998 Transforming nursing through reflective practice. Blackwell Science, Cambridge

Menzies I E P 1960 A case study in the functioning of social systems as a defence against anxiety. Human Relations 13: 95–121

Nichols K 1993 Psychological care in physical illness, 2nd edn. Chapman & Hall, London, Ch 5, p 108

Rafferty M 1998 Clinical supervision In: Barnes E (ed) Face to face with distress. Butterworth Heinemann, London

Savage J 1995 Emotional and physical aspects of care. In: Nursing intimacy, an ethnographic approach to nurse-patient interactions. Scutari, London, Ch 6, p 53

Winnicott D W 1960 Casework and mental illness. In: The maturational process and the facilitating environment. Hogarth, London

Section 2

Life span, emotional development and sexuality

Introduction

Introduction

In Section 1 sexuality was discussed in relation to clinical practice and the need for practitioners to be aware of the disruptions and anxieties often experienced by people in health and illness. In this section, attention is turned to developmental issues that are relevant and that should shape our styles of work. Chapter 7 focuses on the key concepts that apply to the processes involved in the emergence of individuality, and is concerned with both normal development and the difficulties people may encounter during their life span. This developmental approach is crucial to clinical work, which is about understanding how things are for an individual. The perspective represents a crucial shift in the way development is considered (Sroufe & Rutter 1984, Cicchetti 1989, Rutter 1996). There has been a move away from concentration on a universal progression through a series of predetermined stages (such as Freud's psychosexual stages and Piaget's cognitive levels), towards the dynamic mechanisms operating over time in the ways in which individuals deal with adaptations and maladaptations. The emphasis is now on understanding how the complex mix of continuities and change comes about, and how this gives rise to individuality. Chapter 7, therefore, starts with a discussion of just what this developing individuality is. What does the notion of a 'person' involve and how does the process of development operate?

Chapter 8 looks at some of the manifold ways in which development involves an interplay between nature and nurture. Over recent years it has come to be appreciated that human characteristics cannot be divided into those that are genetic and those due to upbringing. Rather, individuality results from a dynamic process involving both the universals of biological maturation and the variations and changes brought about by the interplay of genes and environment. Chapter 8 seeks to give a flavour of the exciting findings in this field as well as pointing to the many important implications for clinical practice.

Chapter 9 considers the specifics of becoming a sexual person and discusses how this fits in to the overall pattern of sexual relationships and social functioning. It emphasizes the different facets of sexuality – the development of the concept of being male or female; patterns of ideas on what is acceptably 'masculine' or 'feminine' in styles of behaviour; the growth of sexual urges; emergence of selective sexual relationships; and the growth of love for another person.

Chapter 10 tells the story of what is involved in social relationships as they operate across a life span, and how those in adulthood derive from transitions and experiences in earlier life. Again, the message is that both change and continuity are involved.

Chapter 11 picks up the importance of experiences in adult life in shaping individuality. Traditional developmental textbooks in years gone by tended to assume that development ceased once physical growth was complete. We now know that is not so; many key experiences do not take place until adulthood. Thus, leaving home, establishing a work career, developing a sexual relationship, becoming a parent and experiencing bereavement usually first take place in the years after puberty. Chapter 11 discusses their impact and how responses to these adult experiences may be shaped by what has occurred during the years of childhood and adolescence

Chapter 12 deals with the impact of illness on sexuality. It notes that the impact incorporates not just the changes brought about by the illness itself but the consequences of the experience of illness on a person's self-concept and on their relationships with other people.

REFERENCES

Cicchetti D 1989 Developmental psychopathology: Past, present and future. In: Cicchetti D (ed) The emergence of a discipline. Rochester Symposium on Developmental Psychopathology. Erlbaum, Hillsdale, N J Vol 1, pp 1–12

Rutter M 1996 Developmental psychopathology: concepts and prospects. In: Lenzenweger M F, Haugaard J J (eds) Frontiers of developmental psychopathology. Oxford University Press, Oxford, pp 209–237

Sroufe L A, Rutter M 1984 The domain of developmental psychopathology. Child Development 55: 17–29

7

The development of a person

Marjorie Rutter

KEY ISSUES

- Domains of development are both separate and interconnected
- Development involves both change and continuity
- Individual differences operate from the outset but are further shaped by experiences
- Important experiences are outside as well as inside the family
- People attribute meaning to their experiences and this meaning influences the impact
- Social context alters meaning
- Experiences change us as people, and early experiences shape later experiences and people's responses to them

INTRODUCTION

The person that we become as an adult involves at least three different components:

1. patterns of competence and capacities
2. habitual styles of behaviour
3. self-concept.

1. People vary in their social skills; their ability to interest and engage other people; their sensitivity and responsivity to social cues and signals; their ability to confide and to share feelings; their capacity to make committed relationships and their facility for trusting and engendering trust in others.

2. Similarly, there are marked individual differences in social styles. Some people are gregarious and enjoy social occasions; others are much more self-contained and content with their own company; still others would like to join in but are held back by their shyness and anxiety. Some interact with humour and warmth; others habitually provoke, confront and antagonise. Some are intellectually curious, loving the challenge of new ideas; others are less adventurous, preferring to stick with the familiar.

3. In a way, the third component, the self-concept, is the one that is most distinctively human. We are not only social beings, we are thinking, feeling beings. Our capacity for language and for thinking means that we actively process all our experiences. We think about what happens to us and we conceptualize, label and remember those experiences in particular ways. We look ahead into the future, as well as looking back into the past. In so doing, we develop ideas about ourselves and about our relationships. Some people gain a concept of themselves as effective, problem-solving individuals able to cope with change and challenge; others perceive themselves as helpless and at the mercy of fate. Some assume that other people will naturally like them; others expect rejection, rebuffs and humiliation. The importance of these self-concepts lies in the fact that they shape both our feelings about ourselves and the ways in which we react to new experiences and new relationships.

This chapter outlines how personal identity emerges through several related developmental processes.

Developmental domains are separate but interconnected

It is obvious to all of us that human functioning does not develop as one piece. We all know individuals who are academically clever but socially inept, or who are well developed physically but also appear emotionally immature. Similarly, research findings tell us that the factors that influence intellectual growth are not quite the same as those that impinge on social relationships or behaviour (Rutter & Rutter 1993). Active learning experiences and rich environmental interchange are particularly important for intellectual development, and a warm, loving family is vital for the development of social relationships. Nevertheless there are important interconnections between domains. Children who are severely delayed in language acquisition are more likely than other children to experience social problems. Children learn better at school when they have a teacher who is positive and encouraging and shows that she likes them. In thinking about developmental processes, we need to recognise both the separateness and the interconnections between different facets of functioning.

Change and continuity

Development is all about change and it would be absurd to expect stability and consistency. The progression to walking, the emergence of language and the transition of puberty all speak to the massive extent of change. On the other hand, development also gradually brings about a coherence of functioning and an individuality in its expression. On the whole, adults do tend to behave and think in moderately consistent ways across situations and over time. Moreover, they develop a moderately consistent picture of themselves as a particular sort of person.

But that consistency is only moderate and we need to appreciate the features that bring about change and discontinuity. Three factors are crucial.

1. Our internal biological state is influential. People behave differently when they are ill or intoxicated or depressed.

2. Social circumstances influence whether individual propensities are translated into particular behaviours. For example, this is evident in the physical and sexual violence directed at innocent individuals as part of civil conflict or war, or the group behaviour of some football crowds.

3. People often think that experiences bring about change; although they may, experiences usually tend to make people more like they were before. Stress usually enhances pre-existing characteristics. If someone has a history of successful coping, further bad experiences are likely to draw on those strengths, and thereby enhance them. If, on the other hand, a person generally sees challenges as dispiriting sources of yet another likely failure, life stresses will probably increase their sense of helplessness and low self-worth.

When then do experiences result in change? The answer is, when they provide a marked discontinuity with the past. A bad failure at something felt to be really important can destroy a person's self-confidence, as in the break-up of a long-standing love relationship, not so much from the loss itself but from the sense of personal inadequacy that it may create. Conversely, someone from a seriously discordant background who, against all odds, makes a lasting, trusting, confiding love relationship may came to view themselves much more positively and start to deal with life challenges with a sense of efficacy.

Individual differences

The temperamental features of babies are immensely varied, and biological influences play a considerable role in that individuality. Furthermore, these individual differences affect how other people respond to the child. Some children are easier to love than others. In this way, initial differences serve to evoke differences in experiences (see Chapter 8). These experiences, in turn, will influence the course of temperamental development and the ways in which differences develop into personality features.

Experiences inside and outside the family

Until relatively recently, people tended to think about experiences largely in terms of the effects being brought about by being reared in particular sorts of families – affluent or poor, discordant or harmonious, punitive or permissive. Family-wide influences are important but it has become clear that they tend to impinge on different children in different ways. One child may get drawn into family conflict, whereas another remains outside the hostilities; one is consistently favoured, while another is scapegoated. These individual differences within the family matter as least as much as differences among families. However, studies have shown that many important experiences occur outside the family – in the peer group, at school, or in the community. These, too, affect people's development.

Attribution of meaning

Experiences do not act on a passive organism. We actively process experiences, thinking about their meaning and responding differently according to the meaning attributed. For example, clinic staff were surprised when a young woman, who had just been made redundant, arrived looking particularly happy and relaxed. For her, redundancy meant the release from a boring, mundane job she hoped to replace with something more interesting and challenging. The loss of income and security were not so important. For someone else the reverse might be true.

The meaning of experiences may also change over time as social attitudes change. Thus, in the early years of this century, being an illegitimate child was a social disgrace and often meant being unwanted and brought up in unsupported circumstances. This situation carried with it substantial risks for psychological development. By contrast, in the UK today over a third of babies are born out of wedlock but many are much wanted and are being brought up by two parents who are living together but have chosen not to marry. There is not the same stigma and not the same risk.

In many industrialised societies, teenage parenthood constitutes a substantial risk factor for both the marriage (or cohabiting relationship) and the offspring. That is unlikely to apply to groups where arranged marriages in adolescence are the norm and when early childbearing is expected in order to 'prove' fertility and to provide heirs.

It has also been found that stressful experiences can be strengthening rather than damaging if the person copes successfully. Thus, Elder (1979) found that older children who had to take on family responsibilities during the economic depression of the 1930s, and who managed these well, emerged strengthened. By contrast, younger children in the same situation who were less able to cope were more likely to be affected adversely.

Social context alters meaning

The examples already given illustrate the importance of social and cultural context. The issues are crucially important for all of us working in a multi-ethnic, multi-cultural society, but three further points warrant emphasis:

1. We need to be aware that the ways in which we think about cultural and ethnic differences may not coincide with the ways in which other people think about themselves. For example, West Indian parents were delighted when their adolescent daughter was due to see a doctor from Jamaica who had come to London for further training. The daughter, on the other hand, was very fed up that she had to be dealt with by a 'foreigner'. For her, being 'black' was an important part of her identity but being West Indian was not. She was a Londoner and thought of herself as such. Similarly, for many people from the Asian subcontinent, ethnicity is of little or no importance but religion is crucial.

2. A further consideration is that many people have multiple cultural ties (see Case study 7.1). Intermarriage between ethnic groups is becoming increasingly common and, in addition, identities may be self-defined in terms of all sorts of features other than ethnicity (Modood et al 1997). This may mean that people get caught up in within-family clashes about cultural expectations.

Experiences change us as people

If experiences can have a lasting effect (as evidence shows they can) we need to consider how that persistent impact may be mediated and carried forward. We need to understand what is the effect on the organism if we are to know best how to help people. Several different sorts of effects are possible. To begin with there may be physical effects. Experiences are needed to guide brain development. This has been shown most clearly in the role of visual input for fostering the growth and functioning of the part of the brain sustaining visual functioning. That is why it is important to correct early squints in order to maintain binocular vision. Animal studies have also shown how early physical stress leads to alterations in the neuroendocrine system. This effect of experiences on physical structure almost certainly extends more broadly than vision and endocrine glands. The notion of developmental programming (meaning that early experiences 'programme' the

Case study 7.1

Davinda, a 17-year-old school girl came into the room at the family planning clinic frightened and upset. She began by asking if her GP or her parents would be contacted about this visit and she was assured of confidentiality. She then expressed her fears that she was pregnant; the pregnancy test confirmed this. On hearing the result, she gripped the arms of the chair and stared straight in front of her. When I reached over to touch her hand, she was unable to release her grip and continued her icy stare. After a long time she began to tremble and asked if I could help her. She described being in the grip of two cultures, one pulling her to her Asian family traditions with an arranged marriage and early childbearing and parenting, and the other towards Western traditions with her white school friends and their free way of life with the prospect of university and independence. Her father had forbidden her to go out with a sixth-form boy at school and had written to the boy's parents to tell them of plans for Davinda's arranged marriage. He also requested their help to exert pressure on the boy to end the relationship. Her dilemma was intensely distressing. She not only feared she had brought shame on her family and would be rejected, but she would be responsible for the upheaval in her boyfriend's family. She expressed her intense aloneness and felt she did not have a place that belonged to her. She felt unable to choose her future path.

way the body deals with later adaptation) seems to apply to many areas (see Chapter 10 for an example with respect to social relationships).

Alternatively, experiences may lead to altered styles of behaviour that then bring about further effects. For example, if someone learns to respond to stress with heavy drinking, alcohol problems will bring about other consequences. Similarly, if being abused leads to aggressive behaviour, the style of being confrontational and hostile will alter how other people respond to that person.

Another important possibility is that experience may affect how a person thinks about herself, as illustrated in Case studies 7.2 and 7.3.

Early experiences shape later experiences

Finally, early experiences tend to shape both the likelihood of having certain sorts of later experiences and also the style of responding to them. For example, teenage pregnancy may result in dropping out of education (with consequent work and income implications); sporting prowess may open up a range of social as well as career opportunities; an impulsive marriage to escape

Case studies 7.2 and 7.3

Mary had menorrhagia for 7 years. She said she felt ill for at least I week out of every 4, and had lost her job for having taken so much sick leave. She was 38 and did not want any more children, and so decided to have a hysterectomy. However, when I saw her after the operation her reaction was nothing to do with symptom relief but rather with distress that the loss of her womb threatened her identity as a woman, a wife and a lover. She worried what her partner would think of her now and whether the loss of fertility meant a loss of her sexuality.

Peter, at 18 years of age, had an operation for undescended testicles and was told that he might be left infertile. Fourteen years later, at the age of 32 he presented at the clinic with overwhelming anxieties about his difficulties in sustaining heterosexual relationships. For him, the diagnosis of possible infertility had meant uncertainties over whether he could have normal sexual function and this dominated both his view of himself and his approach to relationships.

Reflection point 7.1

Both Peter's and Mary's stories highlight how experiences affect people's patterns of thinking about themselves and the importance for the practitioner of understanding the meaning for each individual person. How would you discuss loss of self-image with a patient?

a stressful family home may bring about a discordant abusive relationship that perpetuates, rather than terminates, chronic social adversity.

In addition, early experiences may be important through their influence on people's susceptibility to later hazards and stress. It is a universal finding that there is enormous individual variation in people's responses to even severe stress and adversity (Rutter 1999). Many factors play a part in bringing about either resilience or vulnerability. These include genetic factors (see Chapter 8) but also they include prior experiences because of their sensitising or steeling effects.

CONCLUSION

The process of development results in a thinking, feeling individual with a particular pattern of social skills, social behaviour and self-concepts. There is no point at which this process comes to an end because personality functioning shows an inherent fluidity (as well as coherence and consistency), and a responsivity to experiences throughout life. Change and continuity are both inherent features and many factors interact in shaping the developmental process. The following chapters consider how this takes place with particular reference to sexuality and social relationships.

BIBLIOGRAPHY

Rutter M, Rutter M 1993 Developing minds: challenge and continuity across the life span. Penguin, London
The importance of this book for practitioners lies in its discussion of the implications of a life span approach, and in its account of how nature and nurture work together over the course of development in making people very similar in some aspects and yet so different in others.

REFERENCES

Elder G H Jr 1979 Historical change in life patterns and personality. In: Baltes P, Brim O G (eds) Life span development and behaviour. Academic Press, New York, Vol 2
Modood T, Berthoud R, Lakey J et al 1997 Ethnic minorities in Britain: diversity and disadvantage. Policy Studies Institute, London
Rutter M 1999 Resilience concepts and findings: implications for family therapy. Journal of Family Therapy 21(2): 119–144
Rutter M, Rutter M 1993 Developing minds: challenge and continuity across the life span. Penguin, London

8

Nature–nurture interplay

Marjorie Rutter

KEY ISSUES

◆ The effects of puberty
◆ The menstrual cycle
◆ The menopause
◆ Susceptibility to environmental hazards
◆ Sensitive phases in development
◆ Parents pass on genes and provide a rearing environment
◆ Effects of an individual's behaviour on other people
◆ Individual shaping and selecting of environments

INTRODUCTION

People often refer to the brain and the mind as if they were alternatives, even though the reality has to be that they represent two facets of the same thing. The workings of the mind take place in the brain and they are reflected in changes in brain functioning. Similarly, emotions involve both bodily changes and feeling states. For example, on seeing a tiger approaching, the physical symptoms of sweating and tachycardia will occur simultaneously with the thought process of fear. Experimental alterations of physiology will produce changes in feelings, but so too, the experimental induction of emotions will lead to hormonal changes. A nice example is provided by a study of a chess game between two closely matched men in which the victor showed a large rise in testosterone but the loser a fall (Mazur et al 1992). This sort of two-way interplay is what biology is all about and, in this chapter, some examples that particularly concern developmental issues are discussed. A distinction is drawn between effects that are universal and those that reflect individual differences; both are important. In puberty the hormonal changes have effects on everyone. The effects on the individual, however, may vary as a result of being unusually early or late in reaching puberty, or of having unusually great or unusually small physical/hormonal changes at this age period.

The effects of puberty

The bodily changes associated with puberty begin when the hypothalamus in the brain signals the pituitary gland to release gonadotrophins into the bloodstream. These hormones, in turn, stimulate the production of oestrogen and androgens from the adrenals and from the ovaries in girls and from the testes in boys. This process begins at about 7–9 years, several years before secondary sexual characteristics appear. The hormone-stimulated growth spurt in girls begins about 10.5 years of age, continuing to about 14 or so. In boys, it begins and finishes some 2 years later. The menarche usually occurs during the mid-phase of the growth spurt, as do nocturnal emissions (wet dreams) in males.

There are both direct and indirect effects of these hormonal changes. The most obvious direct effects are on physique and on sexual characteristics. In girls, there is an increased accumulation of fat, expanding hip dimensions, the growth of breasts and the appearance of pubic and axillary hair. The skin also becomes more greasy and facial acne may appear. In boys, there is an increase in muscle power, a broadening of the shoulders, a more widespread growth of facial and bodily hair than in girls and a greater tendency for a greasy skin and facial acne. In both sexes, but particularly in boys, the production of androgens causes a rise in sexual urges and also some tendency to increased dominance behaviour.

The indirect effects of puberty are many and various. To begin with, there are the reactions to the changes in physique. On the whole, boys welcome them but girls do not. On the other hand, neither sex likes the appearance of blackheads, pimples and acne, and this may cause feelings of unattractiveness and shying away from relationships with the opposite sex. In many societies, including our own, girls are unhappy about getting fatter and by late adolescence about half have dieted, usually unsuccessfully. This dissatisfaction is often accompanied by a loss of confidence and of self-esteem. Most girls spend a lot of time looking in the mirror and evaluating themselves in relation to their peers. Being thin in present-day society is seen as being desirable and the self-categorisation of being fat or heavy is often felt to be unappealing.

Most boys react positively to the changes of puberty. Sometimes first ejaculation may be associated with feelings of guilt if it is linked to masturbation. However, for most boys masturbation no longer carries the threat of damage to health and psyche that it used to have. Brooks-Gunn & Furstenberg (1989) interviewed a small sample of boys about their reaction to first ejaculation and although two-thirds felt a little frightened most had positive responses. However, there was a big difference in response between boys and girls in that most girls had spoken to their mothers about first menstruation, while for boys first ejaculation was a secret event unshared with either peers or father.

Many girls have anxieties about breast development and worry that one breast is becoming larger than the other or friends' breasts are growing much faster. Some mothers encourage their daughters to discuss their feelings about their development, whereas others do not acknowledge any changes, however obvious. Either of these responses may affect their daughter's self-image and feelings about having become a woman (Ussher 1989).

The menarche is a marker for growing up, of the need for independence, and of having become a sexual being. For some girls this is a source of pride and joy but for others it can be a frightening and lonely experience. Myths and taboos about menstruation are prevalent, with terms such as 'curse', 'package of troubles' and 'bloody Mary' very widespread. In some families it is important to conceal periods from males and sanitary wear has to be hidden, emphasising silence and secrecy. Some girls may persistently present at the clinic with complaints of dysmennorhoea, which may be associated with underlying anxieties that are difficult to express, concerning the transition to sexuality and womanhood. There may be worries about unpleasant odours, the loss of blood and concerns over the body becoming out of control. The feelings girls have as they go through puberty will be influenced by their own self-esteem and body image as well as by the relationships within their family, and with peers and teachers. The mother–daughter relationship is influential in the formation of the girl's perception of femininity and womanhood. If the mother is embarrassed, her daughter may pick up negative feelings and become anxious herself. Mothers can sometimes be jealous of their daughters' emerging sexuality, which may emphasise their own increasing age or opportunities that were never fulfilled. A mother who is uncertain of her own value as a woman will not provide a good model for her daughter. On the other hand, if she is warm and sensitive and is perceived by her daughter as a successful sexual woman, then it is more likely that her daughter will develop a happy sexual identity herself.

Adolescence is also associated with an increase in a range of problems, including eating disorders, depression, suicidal behaviour, antisocial activities, and drug/alcohol problems. It seems unlikely that the hormonal changes of puberty play a direct stimulating role in their occurrence but, as with the other responses to puberty, there may be indirect effects.

Unusually early puberty

As with other developmental transitions, there is huge individual variation in the age at which children reach puberty. Some girls have their menarche at age 9 years and others not until 14 years. The very fact of being out-of-step with other children can be a source of anxiety and embarrassment. It is not very easy being the only girl in the primary school class having periods. The early putting on of weight before this is happening with others may have adverse effects on self-image and/or lead to troublesome dieting and preoccupation with body shape. There may also be consequences that derive from other people's reactions. Sexual advances may come early to girls reaching puberty before their peers. Also, early maturity may lead girls to become part of an older peer group which, in turn, may increase the likelihood of engaging in truancy, heavy drinking, drug taking and unruly behaviour. Research findings have shown the reality of these disadvantageous effects of early puberty in girls but have also shown that they are mediated by the older peer group (Caspi & Moffit 1991). The stimulus is physical but the immediate causal mechanism is social.

The menstrual cycle

The menstrual cycle well illustrates some of the key features of nature–nurture interplay. To begin with, the onset (the menarche) represents a universal, biological transition in females, an event controlled by the genes. It introduces cyclical hormonal changes that constitute a break with earlier childhood. Although the occurrence of the menarche is universal, there are huge individual differences in its timing, in the psychological reactions to the changes of puberty and in the psychological reactions to the changes within the cycle. The first two features have already been discussed and here we consider the third in the context of the concept of premenstrual tension (PMT).

The menstrual cycle produces a whole range of physical and emotional effects which vary in their impact from one woman to another, from one cycle to another, and from one time of life to another. The term 'premenstrual tension', while reflecting how it is felt, has now been replaced in some medical circles by the term 'premenstrual syndrome', which implies an illness. There is controversy about this terminology which reflects some of the unease of the negative labels that have been attached to it, such as 'it's her bitchy time – just ignore her', or 'she's neurotic' or 'going off her nut'. Because there is some disagreement within the medical profession over the definition, women may find it difficult to have their symptoms acknowledged as valid.

The presence of the hormone progesterone, which enters the bloodstream after ovulation, takes place on about day 14 of the menstrual cycle. This gives rise to physical changes that are most noticeable from mid-cycle, until the next period begins 14 days later. Associated physical symptoms include breast swelling, abdominal bloating, peripheral oedema, headaches, increase in greasy skin and acne, change in bowel habits, changes in appetite and lack of coordination. There may also be emotional reactions at this time that can give rise to tension, irritability, mood swings, depression, anxiety, restlessness and lethargy. Unquestionably, hormonal changes bring about physical changes but the question is whether the hormones directly cause the negative emotions. Strong claims have been made that they do (Dalton 1984). However, other studies have shown that the association is rather weak and that, for the most part, women who show negative emotions have other stresses and anxieties in their lives (Bancroft 1989). Clare (1983) also found that women presenting with PMT were more likely than other women to complain of interpersonal conflicts and marital disharmony and to show higher anxiety levels.

Women's experiences regarding the meaning of their menstruation appear to be influential. There are many different links between menstruation, pain, fear, sex, dirt and gender, as shown in Mary's story.

Case study 8.1

Mary came to the clinic complaining of increasing tension and irritability before her period. She said she felt out of control and her husband was 'going mad'. She said, 'I've always had trouble with my periods from day one.' She recalled her first day when she went to the toilet at her primary school and saw blood on her knickers. She felt frightened and started to scream so that the girl in the next cubicle ran to get a teacher. When the teacher arrived she said 'Get up and stop being silly – you're behaving like a baby. You're a big girl now.' She was taken to the medical room and given a sanitary pad and was told she was making a fuss about something that was completely normal – 'it's just your period'. The teacher sent her home early but Mary felt the blood was going to pour down her legs so sat on a park bench for an hour until she finally got courage to go home. Her mother was matter-of-fact – 'Everyone gets periods – you'll get used to it', and so Mary was left on her own fearing something was wrong. She was frightened to go to school in case other children found out. She was sure this had never happened to anyone else. Eventually she did confide in her best friend whose older sister explained what it was all about. Mary said, 'I've always had trouble from that day to this. I've never had any help but I hope you can help me now.'

> ## Reflection point 8.1
>
> Mary was able to talk about her anger with the teacher and her mother which she had never expressed before. How would you handle a patient's anger about events in the past?

Laws (1990) reported that many women focus on the physical symptoms rather than acknowledging the underlying distress. It is certainly evident in the clinical setting that many women present with physical complaints and when these are taken at face value the hidden distress may never be identified. Often it can be helpful to directly ask about anxieties or distress in their lives.

Many women from different cultures also have negative feelings about their periods. They consider that they are unclean whilst menstruating and use such words as 'Avadi' ('polluted' in India) and 'Kotoran' ('dirt' in Java) (Laws 1990). Men's attitudes can affect how women feel about their menstruation. Boys use taunting and jokey words about menstruation such as 'jam sandwich', or 'jam roll' referring to sanitary pads. Periods may have to be kept secret within the family. Some girls are told 'Never let your brother see this, whatever you do' (Laws 1990). During menstruation men may also give negative responses to their partners when the idea of intercourse at that time is dirty and disgusting. Women can also be described as 'going mad' or 'off the hinge' at this time, which may give rise to anxieties about their mental state.

Views on PMT remain somewhat divided (Walker 1997). The possibility of direct hormonal effects cannot be completely ruled out but it seems highly likely that this is not the whole story. Psychological reactions to the cyclical changes need to be considered in relation to other aspects of a woman's emotional state, to past experiences and to her current social situation.

The menopause

Nature–nurture interplay in relation to the menopause closely parallels that already discussed in relation to puberty and PMT. Its occurrence is a biological universal but there are marked individual differences in both timing and reactions to it.

The menopause refers to the final menstrual period, whereas the perimenopause or climacteric describes the time leading up to and just after the last period which lasts, on average, about 5 years. During this time ovarian production of oestrogen declines and with this decline come bodily changes which may be unpleasant. The menopause commonly occurs between 45 and

58 years of age but can begin earlier than this. A menopause prior to age forty is described as an early menopause. These women are particularly vulnerable to both physical and psychological symptoms (Box 8.1).

The effects of these physical symptoms may cause distress and confusion. Some women say, 'I feel different – I don't understand what is happening to me.' Many women experience a drop in the capacity for physical exercise and complain of tiredness.

The psychological symptoms of the menopause are well documented. Women report feelings of loss of confidence, sadness, depression and being worthless. Are these symptoms in direct response to loss of oestrogen or are there other factors involved? We need to ask what is the meaning of the experience of the menopause for each woman.

For some women who have prized their youthfulness and energy, this change tends to lower their self-confidence and self-esteem and reminds them of getting old. There can be feelings of sadness surrounding the loss of children who are becoming independent and leaving home. Many women feel they do not have a role in life when their children have gone. They may have been dependent on their children for a raison d'etre, and now feel life does not have much to offer. They may become depressed and feel useless and boring. Relationships with teenage children may be difficult at this time, with confrontations and rows that are upsetting. There may be anxieties about becoming less attractive and losing their partner to another woman, feelings that may give rise to self-doubt and a flurry of activity for beauty treatments, diets and the like. Being fertile is frequently felt to be synonymous with being feminine, sexual and attractive, and when these are gone women may feel diminished and of less value.

Other stressful events, coinciding with the menopause, such as death or illness of parents and friends, can induce feelings of sadness and depression. For the woman this may induce anger when the burden of looking after ill or ageing parents robs her of the freedom she was expecting when her children left home. Another response may be a feeling of loneliness: 'I don't think it's

---

Box 8.1 Body changes due to oestrogen loss

◆ Narrowing of the vagina, which becomes drier and less elastic with an increased risk of soreness.

◆ Hot flushes and sweats may be an embarrassing problem and affect sleep.

◆ A gradual decline in muscle tone.

◆ A loss of bone density.

◆ An increase in the risk of heart disease.

my menopause that's the problem. My mother died a few months ago and I'm missing her so much. We've always been close and I could talk to her about anything. I think I've always relied on her a lot. I really need someone who will understand how I feel.'

Men, too, may have their own difficulties at this time. Problems with work and career, and financial worries can loom large as retirement or the fear of redundancy approaches. There may be fears about loss of sexual drive and potency. Changing self-image can be difficult with weight gain and loss of physical fitness.

The hopes and expectations that people bring to events will be influential in their negotiation of the event. For many, it is seen as a time of new challenges, rich freedoms and opportunities. A patient described her hopes in this way: 'I look on it as a change for the better. My husband and I have just planned a wonderful holiday in Spain. No children to bother about – we'll just please ourselves. We'll be free for the first time in years, just the two of us again.' For others, it may feel like a closing down, giving rise to anxiety, an uncertainty about the future and the feeling of 'downhill all the way'.

There are many myths and stereotypes about the menopause and a common one is that it means that sexuality will fade out and emotional problems will arise. For some women the view that when you have reached a certain age you are 'past it' is a relief when intercourse has never been welcomed or enjoyed. Another finding is that sex is bound up with fertility and once this has gone then sex is not for personal pleasure. Sexuality and the menopause are discussed in Chapter 11.

The menopause is often described as a Western culture-bound syndrome which mainly affects white women of European origin, (Hunter 1990). In cultures where the menopause and older age bring increased status and fewer burdens it seems there are no adverse psychological effects. The menopause is not stressful for everyone and for those who present with distress it is important to look at what has gone before. It may be that there have been unhappy unfulfilling relationships and low self-esteem which are now presenting as menopausal difficulties.

Other people's responses are especially influential and many women who are in a relationship during this time find that their partner does not understand the symptoms. One man said, 'I just couldn't understand what was happening to my wife. She was always tired and depressed and didn't want to have sex. I felt that we weren't close anymore. I couldn't bear it any longer and I insisted we had a talk about things and she finally told me what it was all about. I was so relieved to know and since then we've been a lot closer.'

To a major extent, the biological changes associated with the menopause, and with other aspects of the ageing process are universal and inevitable. But they are modifiable, as exemplified by the powerful effects of hormone replacement therapy (HRT) and continuing vigorous exercise. However, the psychological effects of the menopause are not relieved by HRT and in order to understand these it is crucial to consider the meaning for the person in her social setting.

Susceptibility to environmental hazards

Studies have shown an enormous individual variation in how people respond to stress and adversity (Rutter 1999). Many factors play a part in determining susceptibility to environmental hazards. These include:

1. previous adverse experiences that have left the person damaged and more sensitive to later stresses
2. a lack of protective influences or the presence of additional adversities at the time
3. a genetic vulnerability.

The first of these is illustrated by Marguerite's case.

Case study 8.2

Marguerite had recently been given bad news that she could no longer continue her fertility treatment because she was too old. She had been trying to conceive for 6 years and since having the news felt she could no longer cope. She stayed at home wandering round the house or staring out of the window and had uncontrollable tears when her neighbour told her she was pregnant. She said, 'Sometimes I hear a baby crying but I know I'm never going to have my baby now.' As she said this, tears of grief began and she could not speak for a long time. Later she said, 'I did have a baby a long time ago but it was so awful I never thought of that baby.'

Marguerite had become pregnant at 15 when her mother was in a hospice dying of breast cancer. When her distraught father was told about the pregnancy he called Marguerite wicked and said he would never forgive her for what she had done. She was an evil girl to cause so much grief at this time and he did not wish to be in the same house with her. Marguerite wanted to ask forgiveness of her mother, but death came quickly and it was too late for Marguerite.

She went through the termination alone and afterwards was sent to live with her grandmother. Marguerite did not know whether her grandmother knew the reason for her being sent away and the experience was unspeakable for her and had remained so until now. The experience of the events surrounding this pregnancy were so devastating that she never acknowledged or grieved the loss and it was only now that her future without a child evoked the loss.

The point about the current situation is that the social context influences the psychological meaning of the experiences and hence the threat to well-being that is involved. If acute stress derives out of chronic difficulties, if it hits a sensitive spot of previously established sensitivities, or if it leads to a train of negative circumstances, the psychological risks will be greater. Conversely, if the acute event occurs against a background of harmony, or if there is strong social support, damage is less likely. Good experiences are not, in themselves, particularly protective but they are helpful if they counteract or neutralise stresses. Thus, a good new friendship may alleviate the pain of loss of an old friendship, and a problem with one aspect of work may be counterbalanced by particular success in another aspect.

The importance of genetic vulnerability has become increasingly evident in recent years. At one time it used to be thought that what was inherited was an increased direct risk of a particular disorder but it has become apparent that, with the exception of unusual single gene disorders, that is not the way genetic risks operate in relation to complex behaviours that are influenced by both genetic and environmental factors. First, it is usual for several (sometimes many) genes to be involved. Each gene has only quite a small effect; the main risks derive from several genes acting together. Moreover, the risks lie as much in the lack of protective genes as in the presence of susceptibility genes. Second, in most cases the genes exert their influence on normal traits rather than on diseases or disorders as such. Thus, in the psychosocial arena they may act on temperamental features such as emotionality or impulsivity. Third, one of the main ways in which genes bring about their effects is through influences on susceptibility to environmental stressors. Thus it has been found that genes affect people's vulnerability to malaria, to the heart risks associated with smoking and to allergens in the atmosphere. Similarly it seems that they affect vulnerability to both acute stress and chronic adversity. Often, it is the individuals who carry genetic risks who are the most likely to be damaged by environmental hazards.

Sensitive phases in development

One particular feature influencing sensitivity to environmental hazards is maturity. It is not that there is any one age when the risks are greatest, but rather that each developmental phase is more risky for some experiences and less risky for others. For example, babies and older children are less at risk from separation experiences than are toddlers. Babies are less vulnerable because they have not yet developed selective attachment relationships with their parents; older children are protected because they have learned to maintain relationships during separation. Conversely, grief reactions following bereavement tend to be more marked during adolescence than during earlier childhood because as children grow older their abilities to look back and look forwards in time are greater and because of that, the experience of loss may involve extra long-term meaning.

Parents passing on genes and providing a rearing environment

When we find that our patients have suffered damaging experiences in their upbringing there is a natural tendency to assume that those experiences have caused the problems with which they are presenting at the clinic. In part, that may well be the case. There is good evidence that persisting bad experiences can create important psychological risks. It is important, however, to appreciate that the rearing environment will ordinarily have been provided by biological parents who have also passed on their genes. If the parents' failures in parenting derived from their own problems (such as depression or alcoholism), and if genetic influences played some part in the origins of those problems, the difficulties of the next generation may stem from their inherited genetic susceptibilities as well as from their bad experiences. Also, as we have seen, genetic risks operate in part in making people *more* vulnerable to adverse environments. In addition, as we discuss in the next two chapters, genetically influenced personal characteristics exert some of their effects through their role in bringing about exposure to risk environments.

Effects of an individual's behaviour on other people

Humans are social beings, as discussed in Chapter 10, and this means that their social relationships are a crucial part of life. It also means that the most important experiences concern those relationships. Throughout life the main risks do not derive from events such as dog bites or accidents, but rather from personal rebuffs, rejections and humiliations or from interpersonal discord and conflict. All these social experiences involve the individual as well as other people and that implies that their own behaviour is likely to have contributed to eliciting or contributing positive or negative effects from others. Robins (1967), in her classic study following antisocial boys into middle age, showed that they were many times more likely than other boys to have fallen out with their friends, to have been divorced at least twice and to lack supportive relationships. It is easy to see how this happens. Quarrelsome, aggressive, disruptive behaviour makes it more difficult to make and maintain friendships and love relationships.

This powerful effect also applies to interactions with professionals and we need to appreciate how some patients 'get under our skin' and elicit negative responses which carry the danger of reinforcing the patient's negative way of behaving (see Case study 8.3).

Case study 8.3

Mr and Mrs Norris were attending a fertility clinic for in vitro fertilisation. Their names had been on the waiting list for about 9 months when Mr Norris, a university lecturer, made an appointment to see the counsellor on his own. When he came in he did not respond to the greeting or the handshake and when asked to take a seat moved the chair back as far as possible. When asked, 'Perhaps you could tell me why you have come today?' he immediately responded in a loud voice that he was extremely disappointed and angry about the care he was getting.

He continued, 'We thought it would be different here but it's just as bad as the other places we've been to. We've been everywhere and we never get anywhere. You're seen once and nobody really explains the problem and then you just sit and wait. I've been reading all the latest medical journals on sperm problems – I should think I know more than the doctor now.'

Mr Norris's behaviour was powerful, angry and contemptuous and he failed to acknowledge that he had already had two consultations with the doctor. It was difficult to reach Mr Norris's distress because his aggressive behaviour put up an enormous barrier which he did not wish to acknowledge but which gave rise to successive episodes of feeling uncared for and unsupported.

These effects may also stem from physical characteristics and from the prejudices that they engender. It is a regrettably widespread feature of human functioning that group membership is used (often unconsciously) to infer personal qualities. All of us have got to be aware that we are likely, on occasions, to make wrong assumptions about a client because of their gender, religion, ethnicity, style of dress, accent or physical appearance. That is what discrimination is all about and it is something that we are all prone to feel, however much we wish to avoid it. It is also important to recognise this tendency to prejudice even when it has a solid factual basis at a group level. For example, males are much more likely than females to engage in violent crime but it would be quite wrong to assume that an individual man will be violent; most men are non-violent. Similarly, in our society, young people of Asian background do better than average educationally and those from a Turkish Cypriot background do somewhat worse. But that does not mean that all Asians are academic or that all Turkish Cypriots have failed educationally. We need to take care that we respond to people as they are and not on the basis of unwarranted assumptions that derive from their appearance or their background.

There are two other features that we need to note about the effects of individual behaviour on other people. First, this often leads to different children in the same family being treated differently (see Case study 8.4).

> ### Case study 8.4
>
> Mrs Burley suffered from recurrent depression and when she was feeling low she would get very irritable and bad tempered, shouting at her husband and the children. She was worried that this seemed to be dividing the family. Her son, who was a rather assertive boy, usually shouted back and often behaved defiantly or had a tantrum. This infuriated his mother who felt he showed no sympathy for her stressed state. As a result he usually became a target of her anger and Mrs Burley was concerned she was coming to scapegoat him. By contrast, the younger daughter withdrew, went quiet and kept out of the way. The mother often felt guilty about her outbursts and would burst into tears, hugging and cuddling her daughter for comfort. As a consequence the girl became concerned to stay close to her mother in case she was needed. Mrs Burley expressed worries that this was resulting in her daughter getting caught up in her depression and that this was not good for her.

The second feature is the tendency, well described by Patterson (1982), for cycles of negative interchange to develop in some families, but not others. The father yells at one child, the mother intervenes to criticise her husband, he then shouts abuse telling her to keep out of it, another child then enters the quarrel and within minutes everyone is shouting at everyone else. By contrast, in other families, when father yells, the wife is skilled at diverting and in turning the interaction into some more positive activity.

Individual shaping and selecting of environments

Robins' (1967) study illustrated not only immediate effects of people's behaviour on others' responses, but also long-term consequences. Antisocial boys truanted and dropped out of school, left without educational credentials, went to dead-end unskilled jobs, walked out of those jobs when difficulties developed and thereby had rates of unemployment far above those in the general population. Similarly, Quinton et al (1993) described how chains of events led girls from gross family discord to impulsive sexual relationships with antisocial boys, to a teenage pregnancy and then to an unhappy, unsupporting cohabiting relationship, followed by difficulties in parenting their own children and breakup of the relationship. In both studies, people's styles of behaviour served to bring about further damaging experiences. This is usually considered as shaping and selecting effects on experiences but we need to appreciate that such effects do not necessarily result from deliberate choices. Girls may not want a violent, delinquent partner but still land up with someone like that because they put themselves in social situations in which those are the sorts of boys they meet; for example Samantha's story (Case study 8.5).

> **Case study 8.5**
>
> Samantha had been separated from her siblings, was taken into care when aged 3, and she scarcely remembered her parents. Up to the age of 16 she had been in five different homes. At 16 she became pregnant and went to live with her boyfriend who was unemployed. They had very little money and sometimes went hungry. However, Samantha was overjoyed when the baby arrived and did her best to look after her. She tried very hard to be a good mother but her boyfriend couldn't cope with trying to look after them both, said he couldn't stand the baby's screaming and so left her for another girl. The baby became neglected and was taken into care. Samantha subsequently had several boyfriends in quick succession and contracted a sexually transmitted infection. At this point she was referred to the family planning clinic where she was helped to start a method of contraception and negotiate safe sex. Unfortunately she did not use either effectively and became pregnant again but decided to have a termination of pregnancy as her boyfriend 'didn't want to know'. Following the termination she took the injectable contraceptive for 6 months until she met an older man. At her next clinic visit Samantha decided not to have the next injection because she and her new partner wanted to have a baby. Although Samantha's first child was still in care she was sure she would be able to cope this time with the help of her older partner. She talked about their dreams and plans for the future. Samantha did become pregnant again but towards the end of the pregnancy the relationship broke up and again Samantha was left unsupported with another child. She returned to the clinic after the birth for another injection but continued to hope that one day she would have her own family for love and support.

CONCLUSION

In this chapter we have sought to explain some of the many ways in which individual characteristics and personal experiences work together to bring about either adaptive or maladaptive life trajectories. Personality is not controlled by genes or set by experiences in the pre-school years but both may have long-term effects through the chains of circumstances they set in motion. The clinical challenge in considering people's life span developmental course is to understand what seems to have made matters better or worse.

BIBLIOGRAPHY

Laws S K 1990 Issues of blood. Macmillan, London
Ussher J M 1989 The psychology of the female body. Routledge, London
Walker A E 1997 The menstrual cycle. Routledge, London

REFERENCES

Bancroft J 1989 Human sexuality and its problems, 2nd edn. Churchill Livingstone, Edinburgh

Brooks-Gunn J, Furstenberg F F Jr 1989 Adolescent sexual behaviour. American Psychologist 44: 249–257

Caspi A, Moffit T E 1991 Individual differences are accentuated during periods of social change: the sample case of girls at puberty. Journal of Personality and Social Psychology 61: 157–168

Clare A W 1983 Psychiatric and social aspects of premenstrual complaint. Psychological Medicine Monograph Supplement 4: 1–58

Dalton K 1984 The premenstrual syndrome and progesterone therapy, 2nd edn. William Heinemann Medical Books, London

Hunter M 1990 Your menopause. Pandora Press, London

Laws S 1990 Issues of blood. Macmillan, London

Mazur A, Booth A, Dabbs J M 1992 Testosterone and chess competition. Social Psychology Quarterly 55: 70–77

Patterson G 1982 Coercive family process. Castalia, Eugene, Oregon

Quinton D, Pickles A, Maughan B, Rutter M 1993 Partners, peers and pathways: assortative pairing and continuities in conduct disorder. Development and Psychopathology 5: 763–783

Robins L 1967 Deviant children grown up. Williams & Wilkins, Baltimore

Rutter M 1999 Resilience: concepts and findings: implications for family therapy. Journal of Family Therapy 21(2) 119–144

Ussher J M 1989 The psychology of the female body. Routledge, London

Walker A E 1997 The menstrual cycle. Routledge, London

9

Becoming a sexual person

Marjorie Rutter

KEY ISSUES

- ◆ The several facets of sexuality
- ◆ Influences on sexual activities
- ◆ Some features of teenage sexuality
- ◆ Early adulthood
- ◆ Sexuality in the middle and later years

INTRODUCTION

Sexuality is a crucial part of what it is to be human, but it incorporates far more than the sex act. We define ourselves as male or female and act accordingly; we like to appear attractive to others; love relationships are an important part of most people's lives (even if they do not involve sexual activities); and sexual urges are part of our biology. In this chapter we start with a consideration of the multi-faceted nature of sexuality, and then move on to consider some features that are of particular importance in different age periods.

THE SEVERAL FACETS OF SEXUALITY

It is a curious feature of the English language that the word 'sex' is used to cover several rather different concepts.

1. *Biological sex* – the biological features associated with being male or female.

2. *Gender identity* – a person's view of themselves as male or female.

3. *Sex-typical behaviour* – behaviour that, in any given culture, is considered appropriate for one or other sex.

4. *Sexual attractiveness* – as referred to by the adjective 'sexy', is not quite the same as sex-typical behaviour and need not involve any form of sexuality.

5. *Sexual activity* – behaviours that (at least in adults) provide sexual arousal.

6. *Sexual orientation* – a person's preference for a sexual partner of the same or opposite sex.

Ordinarily, there is a confluence among these several facets of sexuality but there are many exceptions.

Biological sex

Normally, biological sex is determined by a gene on the Y-chromosome with consequent effects on the genital organs, secondary sexual characteristics and pattern of hormone production. There are, however, both chromosome anomalies and other medical conditions that lead to discrepant patterns of one sort of another. Thus, an extra X-chromosome (XXY) in males, or a missing X chromosome (X0) in females, has effects on both fertility and physique.

Gender identity

Gender identity is a person's concept of him or herself as male or female, as reflected in the notion of 'I am a boy' or 'I am a girl'. This identity develops early in the pre-school years and rapidly becomes a central part of a person's self-concept. Studies of individuals with some medical condition requiring a change of sex in childhood indicate how difficult it is to alter this identity and also that the experience of being neither entirely male nor entirely female is an exceedingly uncomfortable one. There is not really an acceptable middle identity. Because the origins of gender identity can only be investigated in individuals with some sort of biological anomaly, it has proved difficult to identify the causal processes with any certainty. Until recently, it was thought that the most important factor determining identity is the sex to which the child is assigned at birth and brought up with. However, physical appearance is likely to play a defining role, and recent evidence suggests that prenatal hormones (with their subtle influences on brain structure) may play a greater role than once thought.

Sex-typical behaviour

The categorisation of individuals by gender is an intrinsic part of understanding other people. These sets of beliefs about what is culturally appropriate 'masculine' and 'feminine' behaviour are learned very early in development and play a critical role in children's behaviour. Because, to a substantial extent, they vary across cultures, they are sometimes termed gender stereotypes, implying that they have no biological basis. This is, however, a somewhat misleading over-simplification for several different reasons. To begin with, some behaviours that differentiate males and females in humans do so similarly in a wide range of animal species, making a purely cultural explanation implausible (Maccoby & Jacklin 1980). Also, there are some differences, such as style of throwing a ball, that seem to have a structural basis in part (deriving from the carrying angle of the arm). There is evidence that prenatal hormones have some effects on later behaviour and that there are some (quite minor) differences between the brains of males and females (Gorski 1996). On the other hand, there can be no doubt that cultural pressures play a considerable role in determining the specifics of what is regarded as 'masculine' or 'feminine' in any particular culture. It should be added that concepts of what are appropriate sex-typical behaviours are very wide-ranging – including physical appearance, attitudes and interests, psychological traits, social styles and occupations (Ashmore et al 1986). On the other hand, it is very apparent that the differences within males or females are at least as great as those between the sexes. By no means are all females soft, dainty and nurturing, nor all males strong, independent and risk-taking. Nevertheless, social pressures are such that individuals who deviate from what is expected are often viewed negatively (Golombok & Fivush 1994). As early as the pre-school years, children come to prefer same-sex groups of children with whom to play, and similarly they soon come to select gender-typed toys (even in the face of parental pressures not to do so). Peer pressures to conform to sex-typical behaviour tend to be quite strong (Langlois & Downs 1980). Interestingly, however, the pressure on males to conform tends to be stronger than that on females.

Sexual attractiveness

Sexuality involves how we feel about ourselves and how others feel towards us. Hogan (1980) stated:

> *Sexuality is much more than the sex act. It is the quality of being human; all that we are as men and women, encompassing the most intimate feelings and deepest longings of the heart to find meaningful relationships.*

It is important to most people to be seen by others as attractive and worthy of love. It is not that they are seeking a sexual relationship, or even wanting to arouse sexual feelings, but rather that being attractive to others is an important part of their self-esteem. Interestingly, the concept applies as much to an 80-year-old as to a nubile teenager. Also, this need to be attractive applies as much to males as to females and continues to be important in illness. For example, a man with terminal cancer of the stomach who was emaciated and scarcely recognisable as his former self said to one of his visiting female friends, 'Please move close and hold my hand'. The need to feel attractive and loved is universal. Although physical qualities play some role, facial expressiveness, a lively social style and an interest in others tend to be of considerable importance.

Sexual activities

All infants are curious about their own bodies, taking pleasure in touching and exploring them. Children quickly become aware of how parents regard their genital areas. Is this an acceptable, normal place ('Oh, what a lovely little bottom') or a disreputable one not to be touched or explored ('Stop doing that – its dirty')? By 4 years of age, many children play games such as 'mothers and fathers' or 'doctors and nurses', involving undressing and possibly exploration of genitals. There is a gradual rise in pre-pubertal sex play, although it is sporadic and does not have the intensity or complexity of later sexual behaviour (Rutter 1980). For both sexes, masturbation increases in the years leading up to puberty.

The anatomical differences between boys and girls are relevant for this sex play (Bancroft 1989). The obvious presence, and frequent handling, of the penis and scrotum in boys leads to a positive descriptive vocabulary, with overt peer group interest in genitals. By contrast, many girls are often strikingly unaware of their clitoris, vagina and urethral opening, with these areas remaining untouched and not a subject for discussion. There is also an absence of explicit language, so that female sex organs tend to be referred to in vague ways – such as 'down there' or 'private parts', or through derogatory words such as 'bush', 'man trap', or 'cunt'. As a result, girls may come to fear what they regard as a taboo area of their body. Boys are well aware of penile erections (showing them off to peers in sexual games) but there is no obvious parallel in girls. Accordingly, girls tend to have less awareness of their sex organs. As children pass through puberty, there is a marked upsurge in these sexual activities in three respects:

1. There is a marked increase in sexual urges leading to masturbation and, in boys, to wet dreams, as well as to a rich proliferation in both sexes of sexual fantasies.

2. Sexual curiosity increases with games involving mutual masturbation, boys comparing the size of their erect penises or the strength of their ejaculatory spurt, as well as activities involving the viewing (or, less often, touching) of the sexual areas of the opposite sex.

3. Both boys and girls are likely to want to express their amorous feelings in kissing, caressing and sexual contacts. As always, these will involve a complex mixture of impersonal sexual lust and the expressions of love and affection.

Sexual orientation and love relationships

The beginnings of sexual orientation and of love relationships are evident in middle childhood, well before puberty is firmly established. Nine and 10-year-olds frequently have pin-up pictures of pop stars in their bedroom; boys 'fancy' particular girls at school (and vice versa); there is an interest in sexuality in the media; and boys especially become fascinated by nude and semi-nude pictures of females. During adolescence, same-sex, as well as opposite-sex, 'crushes' are common (especially in girls), even in those who later are exclusively heterosexual. Although the great majority of adults feel and label themselves as definitely homosexual or heterosexual, probably most have some potential within themselves for both. This is evident, for example, in the homosexual activities engaged in (by individuals who are heterosexual in other circumstances) when living in an exclusively same-sex, closed environment, such as a prison or single-sex boarding school.

At first, such early crushes, although feeling intense at the time, do not necessarily involve a conscious desire for sexual activities, and they do not necessarily have the all-encompassing emotional engagement with the other person as an individual. However, they constitute the first beginnings of both sexual lust and love. These two feelings are closely connected (and often difficult for individuals to differentiate) but they are not the same. Both males and females, but perhaps especially males, can feel sexual attraction towards (and even longings for) someone whom they do not know as a person.

Homosexuality

Because heterosexuality is, statistically speaking, so obviously the 'norm', there has been a tendency to view homosexuality as 'deviant' in some way. There has been the assumption that heterosexuality is a biological 'given', unless either there has been a grossly maladaptive upbringing of some kind or some genetic anomaly. It has to be said that the evidence in support of both views is inconclusive. Reports of a so-called gene for homosexuality (based on an atypical sample) have not been confirmed. It is certainly likely that genetic factors play a role in individual differences in sexual orientation (as they do in all human behaviour) but whether they directly cause a particular orientation is more dubious. Occasionally, homosexuality may arise through fears or anxieties over interacting with the opposite sex, and occasionally it may reflect a response to social isolation or alienation. In these instances, it is possible that poor relationships with parents or traumatic sexual experiences may have played a part. It is important to appreciate, however, that sometimes the person's own behaviour (in terms of unusually marked feminine or masculine traits) may have elicited the parental reactions. More usually, individuals become gradually aware of their homosexual orientation as they grow up; often it is not itself a cause of distress to them but there may be considerable embarrassment, unhappiness or even despair over other people's negative reactions. About 1 in 30 women report homosexual experiences in their lifetime (Wellings et al 1994) but, in view of the stigma associated, the true figure may be higher.

Most lesbian women (on the whole, the term 'lesbian' is preferred over the term 'homosexual') view their sexual orientation as an intrinsic part of their being, they do not wish to change, and those who are exclusively lesbian rarely change to heterosexual relationships (although bisexuality is not that uncommon). Some, nevertheless, conceal their lesbianism because they fear being labelled perverted or abnormal. Some women go through long periods of uncertainty over their sexuality, especially if they have married before fully appreciating their homosexuality. Others are anxious about telling their parents, who may be rejecting because of self-blame, because of abhorrence or because they feel that it will cut off their hopes of grandparenthood. When lesbian women have had children in an initial heterosexual relationship, they may fear revealing their sexuality because of concerns over negative responses from husbands and children. Many husbands do indeed react with revulsion but children are more likely to respond positively on the basis of the qualities of the pre-existing loving relationship (if that has been the case) rather than a response to the sexual 'revelation' itself (Bozett 1981).

In the field of clinical practice, issues in relation to lesbianism arise in relation to two main situations. First, practitioners need to avoid assuming that their clients are heterosexual (see Chapter 3). This is particularly so when some homosexuals (male and female) are using heterosexual dating either to avoid stigma or through an attempt to diminish anxieties about their growing awareness of their homosexual orientation (Savin-Williams 1994). Second, practitioners may need to counsel lesbian women seeking donor insemination in order to have a child (or advise on the care of children when a heterosexual marriage breaks up over the mother's lesbianism). In these circumstances, it is important to recognise that the risks do not lie in parental lesbianism as such but rather (as in the case of heterosexual parents) in the personalities of the individuals, their relationship with a partner (if they have one), their attitudes to and behaviour with children, their attitudes towards the opposite sex and their general lifestyle. In other words, each case needs, in the usual way, to be assessed on its merits rather than on the basis of personal prejudice or societal stigma.

INFLUENCES ON SEXUAL ACTIVITIES

Previous social relationships

The essence of sexuality lies in its expression in the context of intimate confiding, loving (or at least affectionate) relationships. Not surprisingly, therefore, a person's previous close relationships, in the form of early attachment relationships and reciprocal friendships, constitute an essential background (and to some extent a basis) for later sexual relationships. Where early relationships have been secure and trusting, it is more likely that the transition to sexual relationships will go smoothly. There will be a continuity with respect to reciprocity and emotional sharing, the newness consisting of the addition of the element of sexuality together with a marked increase in emotional intensity. However, sexuality is likely to be more difficult when these qualities of earlier relationships are lacking. Casual contacts in relationships that tend not to have shared interests and values may lead to risk-taking, impulsive or exploitative sexual behaviour. This situation is common in girls from deprived backgrounds (Pawlby et al 1997a, 1997b).

In addition, however, negotiations may be necessary because of the somewhat different socio-emotional interactive styles of males and females (see Chapter 10). Exclusivity in friendships is more characteristic of girls than boys, and emotional sharing is also more typical. This can lead to a need for adjustments in sexual relationships. A desire for uncommitted sexual 'adventures' is said to be more common in males, and probably is, but it is by no means absent in females, and it is necessary for both partners to be clear what are the rules and expectations of their relationship.

Family

Family influences operate on their children's sexual activities through several rather different routes:

◆ the quality of early attachment relationships will help shape the nature of close friendships
◆ parental attitudes to sexuality and to genitalia will have an impact on how children come to view their own sexual selves
◆ parental attitudes and expectations towards how males and females should behave will have an effect
◆ parental models of sexual and love relationships will be influential
◆ how parents have negotiated conflicts and interpersonal difficulties is important
◆ parental monitoring and supervision will have an influence on the young person's engagement in peer group activities

◆ parental openness and helpfulness in discussing the sexual dilemmas faced by their children are important.

Responsiveness to their needs and feelings is crucial but most young people also want guidance and structure (although not autocratic control). Given the important role of inebriation and drunkenness (together with drug-taking) in removing inhibition and self-control, parental influences on these activities may be as crucial as those on sexuality itself.

Moral values, religion and ethnicity

It is an intrinsic part of development that young people develop moral values, although the specifics of their focus and content will vary according to their temperament, upbringing and sociocultural context. It is a mistake to assume that morality comes only from religion. Adolescents tend to be quite idealistic and usually have firm views on issues such as loyalty and trust in love, as well as other, relationships. Pre-marital sex has now become widely accepted (and expected) in most, although not all, cultures, but most young people express the attitude that it should occur within a relationship that is, at the time, monogamous and committed. That is, serial monogamy is okay but casual promiscuity is not. It has to be said, however, that double standards remain widespread (Lees 1986, Moore & Rosenthal 1992), as reflected in the terms used to describe essentially the same behaviour in males and females; the boy is a 'stud' but the girl is a 'slut'. This dichotomy is particularly marked in some cultures and some religions.

Strong religious beliefs (as distinct from formal church attendance) tend to foster moral values that relate to sexuality. In part they do so because they emphasise the importance of values (this varies greatly, however, among religions), in part because they provide a clear set of rules or guidelines to follow, and in part because of the sanctions they impose (draconian in some religions).

Peer group, youth culture and the media

During the teenage years, peers have a powerful influence on sexual attitudes and behaviour (Hofferth & Hayes 1987). Although young people may well be rebellious in relation to adults, they tend to wish to conform to peer group norms and values (Fishbein & Ajzen 1975). Such norms may act in both positive and negative ways. Moreover, they may derive from personal contacts within groups of friends or from what is perceived to be the youth culture as portrayed in the media. It is quite common for these to pull in different directions. Many of the messages in the media (songs, films and TV) seem to portray hedonistic, violent and self-gratifying sex rather than love relationships.

'Everyone does it', so it must be alright. By contrast, friends may describe how they have negotiated personal relationships in quite different ways. Similarly, school friends may attend family planning clinics together, supporting each other in decisions about contraception. Adolescents face a bewildering mix of messages and standards about how they should behave, and the constructive support of friends and family may be crucial in enabling them to incorporate their options successfully.

Time trends

The last half of the nineteenth century has seen a massive change in sexual activities. Continuing a trend that began much earlier in the century, the age of puberty has fallen progressively so that young people are physically ready for sex at a much earlier age than hitherto. The availability of effective, readily accessible methods of contraception has meant that it has become practical to separate sex for pleasure and sex for procreation. Although there has been a more limited shift in Church teaching on contraception, practice has clearly altered. The birth rate in Catholic Mediterranean countries has fallen dramatically. Partly as a result of an increasing emphasis on women's education and careers, the age of marriage has become much later. Even more dramatically, cohabitation before marriage has become almost the rule in many countries. In addition, an acceptance that sex for pleasure is alright has probably meant a greater willingness to engage in sex play (such as cunnilingus and fellatio) that does not lead directly to procreation. On the other hand, the pandemic of AIDS has led to a greater awareness of the dangers of unprotected sex and has had a constraining influence on homosexuality in certain male settings. Whether or not that will change with the availability of drugs that impede the progress of AIDS remains to be seen.

This greater freedom and permissiveness, however, has not necessarily made sexuality any easier. The same questions about sexual activities arise: Is it voluntary? Is it pleasurable or stressful? Is it a regular or on–off activity? The current controversies over so-called 'date rape' emphasise how easily discrepant expectations can lead to disaster. Once the transition to sexual intercourse has been made, it is likely to be repeated (especially if it is in the course of a committed relationship), and the young person will need quickly to come to decisions on how they wish to handle their sexual life.

SOME FEATURES OF TEENAGE SEXUALITY

In previous sections of this chapter, we have considered the developmental progressions that lead up to teenage sexuality. Here we consider in greater detail a few of the specific considerations.

Love relationships

Early romances may be quite brief, and there may be several in which young people test out relationships and look to same-sex friends for support in making choices about partners. As young people move into their late teens and young adulthood, romantic relationships are likely to become longer lasting, with much exchange of affection, the provision of support in coping with stressful events and a sharing of joint activities. Often, too, these love relationships lead to cohabitation. All of this provides a two-edged sword. On the one hand, the rewards of love are manifold. On the other hand, statistics tell us that the breakdown rate of these cohabiting relationships is high (higher than in marriage), with all the pain of loss that that is likely to entail (not to mention feelings of anger and jealousy).

Contraception

The AIDS pandemic has added to the need for protected sex, and especially for the use of condoms rather than (or in addition to) the contraceptive Pill. This has added several complications to young people's contraceptive practice:

1. Either the responsibility for contraception is placed on the man, or the woman is required to carry male contraceptives.

2. A deliberate planning for sex, rather than allowing it to emerge 'naturally' out of the interaction on the occasion, is implied.

3. There is an implicit message that the girl thinks the boy may carry a disease.

4. It means using a device that (to some extent) is thought to reduce male pleasure.

Not surprisingly, therefore, there are often pressures on girls to engage in unprotected sex. Agreeing to this may mean that she thinks the man is committed to the relationship, thereby giving her a feeling of emotional security (Orbach 1991). Unprotected sex is most likely in a casual encounter (when protection is most needed!) and when sex takes place while under the influence of alcohol.

Contraceptive use is more likely the older the girl is when she first has sex, when this takes place within a committed, stable relationship, and where there is a sense of equality. Girls who feel good about themselves and who feel in control of their lives are more likely to be motivated and effective users of contraception.

Teenage parenthood

In most Western societies, teenage parenthood is a risk indicator (Box 9.1) for both the young people themselves and for their children (Rutter et al 1998).

Box 9.1 Risk factors for teenage parenthood

1. Young people from families where there is discord and poor relationships.
2. A model of early pregnancy in a previous generation.
3. Anti-social risk-taking activities, including taking drugs and alcohol.
4. Low achievement at school.
5. The difficulties of having to cope with being a parent before being properly grown up.
6. Young parents are disadvantaged in education, career and income.

Nevertheless, it should not be assumed that teenage parenthood is always bad, nor is it the case that teenage parenthood always arises in the same way. For a minority, it is a planned and deliberate choice. For others, the pregnancy was unplanned but it occurred in the context of a committed relationship, and the baby becomes loved and wanted. In some cases, it seems that becoming pregnant is a way of showing sexual desirability when a girl lacks status and self-esteem. In yet others, it may be felt to be a means of saving or cementing a relationship (although it rarely serves that purpose well). For some girls, teenage parenthood is a means of escape from an abusing, rejecting home, or a way of punishing controlling, over-protective parents. Occasionally, it is felt to be a method of providing the love for another person (the baby) that the young person lacked in their upbringing. In a few instances, it may reflect ambivalence about sexuality, and in others teenage parenthood reflects an impulsive act.

As we have noted, teenage parenthood carries risks. Nevertheless, these deal with possibilities and not certainties. Follow-up studies show that, in many cases, things can turn out well (Rutter & Rutter 1993), and are more likely to do so if there is good family support and if both young parents can continue with their education. The difficulties, especially in the short-term, include:

◆ feeling of isolation and loneliness because of limited opportunities to join in activities with their peers
◆ anxieties about new heterosexual relationships (because of the disincentive for most men of dating a girl with a child)
◆ feelings of dependency and lack of comfort.

Less has been written about teenage fatherhood but many of the same features apply. In addition, some feel excluded from decision-making about the pregnancy, and problems in providing economic and emotional support are likely to interfere with the lifestyle that they would otherwise be engaging in with their peers.

Termination of pregnancy

When a young person becomes pregnant, the decision to continue or terminate the pregnancy is a major life event, and one that has far-reaching implications for the future. Given the appropriate circumstances, it may be right to keep the baby. On the other hand, abortion can be the best solution for some individuals. When abortion is the choice, it can provide a turning point and an opportunity for reflection. Many teenagers find it difficult to talk to parents about sex and birth control and welcome the new opportunity to get support to enable them to make a decision. Nevertheless, because of society's ambivalent attitudes to abortion, young people frequently present for termination expecting punitive and judgemental attitudes. This may mean that they present their request with unwavering certainty and conviction that hides ambivalent, distressed feelings. Counsellors need to be alert to this possibility (but *not* assume it in the absence of evidence).

After a termination, there may be feelings of loss, guilt, sadness or emptiness. There may also be difficulties with the partner over differences concerning the decision to abort. Occasionally the termination may bring negative attitudes to sex:

◆ worries that the termination means that she is an unworthy person
◆ anxieties about what the operation has done to her body
◆ fears that it may threaten her future fertility
◆ anger over the way she felt she was treated by professionals
◆ fears about future relationships (if this relationship broke up over the pregnancy).

It is necessary to keep these possibilities in perspective. Terminations are now common and most women cope very well without any significant emotional disturbance. In the long run, the outcome is usually good. Nevertheless, termination is a psychologically important event and, in certain adverse circumstances, stresses long forgotten may re-emerge.

Occasionally, unresolved grief may emerge during a subsequent pregnancy or period of infertility or cause distress at the time of delivery. Rarely, there may be fantasies of the fetus at the anniversary of the abortion, at the menopause, or following gynaecological surgery. Practitioners need to be aware of the possibility of unresolved grief giving rise to vulnerabilities many years later. Equally, they should not jump to conclusions before there is evidence that this is what is happening.

EARLY ADULTHOOD

Cohabitation and marriage

Sexual feelings and behaviour do not remain static over the life span, and many people go through a sexually experimental phase, and have a number of partners, before establishing a long-term relationship. Nevertheless, by their 30s most people have established some form of committed cohabiting or marital relationship. To a considerable extent, men and women want the same from such relationships – companionship, intimacy, sexuality and support. But there may be some differences and these require negotiation. On the whole, although there are huge individual differences, men are more likely to attach importance to the frequency of sex and of physical pleasure, whereas women value both the emotional caring and sharing that they can bring. As discussed in Chapter 10, there are some differences (at a group level) in male and female styles of communication and emotional expression. Negotiation in relationships fosters harmony and satisfaction, and the negotiations in relation to sexuality are particularly delicate because of the deep and passionate feelings involved.

Sexuality in pregnancy

The birth of a child is one of the greatest challenges to a couple's relationship and it brings about new experiences that affect both behaviour and sexual feelings. In the ante-natal period, concerns may include:

◆ Will the child be an intruder in the relationship or, in some cases, will it save the relationship?
◆ Will there be support and sharing from the partner or will they feel jealous and excluded?
◆ Will there be anger because the baby restricts the mother's freedom or because feelings of exhaustion will interfere with sex?

Taylor (1992) reported that many men are unprepared both emotionally and intellectually for the birth of their child, and Raphael-Leff (1991) stated that the fact that a woman has a partner need not imply that she is supported. During pregnancy a woman experiences dramatic changes in her physiology, shape and appearance. Concerns about feeling fat, misshapen, unattractive and tired, and having enlarged and heavy breasts, may raise the question, 'Am I attractive enough to love?'

Pregnancy can disrupt the sexual relationship, or may deepen and strengthen it. Many couples feel a sense of well-being and excitement during pregnancy which increases desire and satisfaction, mutual caring, respect, pleasure and intimacy. Some studies report a decrease in sexual activity, which is more marked in the third trimester. This may be due to tiredness, large abdominal size, or pelvic congestion making intercourse seem difficult. Many women fear orgasm will bring on premature labour or that the semen could harm the fetus, and therefore avoid intercourse. When there is a decline in sexual interest by the woman which is not matched by the man, this may provoke guilt and distress in the relationship. It is at these times that other ways of feeling close and achieving sexual satisfaction need to be found.

Pregnancy may bring up painful memories of previous losses, including miscarriage, termination of pregnancy, ectopic pregnancy and cot death. Unexpected sad feelings about family deaths may also be re-awakened. Negative results of a fetal diagnostic test or death of a twin in utero may lead to painful feelings accompanied by fear and apprehension.

Pregnancy is not a universally happy and glorious event, and some pregnancies are surrounded by anxiety and sadness.

Childbirth

The management of labour and delivery can profoundly affect a woman's subsequent feelings about sex. The process of the birth and feelings about sexuality are closely linked. Southern (1994) argued that even if labour does not directly evoke sexual feelings in the woman, it must surely evoke sex. She claimed that women cannot expose themselves to give birth without making this connection. The feelings a woman has about her body after childbirth may be influenced by how she was treated during the birth. Some women feel invaded and not respected, with anxieties about resuming sex after the birth. These feelings may evoke memories of abuse when this has occurred in the past. A traumatic delivery may give rise to fears about damage to the vagina and fears about resuming sex.

For the man, the birth experience may have positive or negative effects. Several writers point out that there is a possibility of psychosexual difficulties for a man witnessing a traumatic delivery. Difficulties about being pressurised to stay, or guilt for not being there, as well as the stress of watching episiotomy and emergency procedures, may have implications for sexuality. Some men feel unable to penetrate the vagina following the trauma and have fantasies of causing more damage. Some men become distressed when the vagina is no longer their domain but becomes invaded by other men. It may appear to be less attractive when the exclusiveness and mystery have been taken away. These examples point to the need for sexuality being recognised as inextricably linked to pregnancy in all its aspects. See Jane's story in Case study 9.1.

Case study 9.1

Jane attended the GP for her post-natal examination. She appeared quiet and sad as she lay down on the couch, and when the doctor attempted to examine her her legs remained drawn up with knees tightly clenched together. Jane began to cry and said she didn't understand why she felt like this. She said that she hadn't been able to make love since the birth of her baby, about 10 weeks ago. The doctor invited her to sit in the chair to talk about her feelings. Jane described feeling let down and disappointed since coming home with the baby. She was finding it difficult to feel enthusiastic and content with things. The baby seemed to be feeding and sleeping well but in spite of this she felt a heavy, dull feeling all the time. When the doctor asked her about the birth she began to cry again and described the experience as disastrous. Everything seemed to go wrong and not as she had planned. She had hoped for a natural birth at home with her midwife but, instead, had had to have an emergency admission to hospital with fetal distress and forceps delivery of the baby. Her distress was compounded by the fact that her husband was abroad on business and could not be contacted in time, so that she was alone for the whole experience. At this point she turned to the doctor, banging her fist on the desk and saying, 'How could he be away at this time?' The doctor and Jane were able to begin to understand some of the feelings that Jane had expressed – her own feelings of failure and disappointment at the birth and the anger towards her husband. In time, she was able to share the feelings with her husband, and they were able to make love again about 6 months later.

Post-natal sexuality

A woman's sexuality following the birth of a baby may include anxieties about perineal pain and soreness as well as a feeling of being less attractive. There may be fantasies about the vagina. For example, 'My vagina must be huge – there were hands and instruments up there trying to get the baby out, I've been stitched up and trussed like a turkey.' It seems that, on the whole, childbearing diminishes sexual activity and enjoyment for about the first year (Robson et al 1981). Moss et al (1986) found that just over a quarter of couples reported gains in their relationship, including sex; however, there were more who experienced negative effects in both relationships and sexuality. Hormonal changes following the birth lower oestrogen levels and raise prolactin levels. These give rise to loss of libido and dry vagina, whilst the physical demands of coping with a new baby can be exhausting. Some women may be completely absorbed in the baby and others talk of 'being in love' with their baby. The experience can be quite shocking when they realise how overwhelming it is. In this situation the partner can feel excluded and may want her to 'mother' him.

Box 9.2 Feelings that impinge on sexuality

◆ prior expectations of 'that wonderful experience' which was dreamed of but not fulfilled
◆ loss of autonomy
◆ relegation of household chores
◆ loss of friends from work days
◆ restrictions imposed by the baby on social life.

Jealousy of intimacy with the baby, or about not being able to share breast-feeding, may occur. Some women gain sexual satisfaction from breast-feeding, and this may engender guilt, particularly when this is linked to reduced sexual interest or arousal.

Van Wert (1991) pointed out that often the problems of changed sexual relationships after childbirth are seen as the woman's fault, i.e. it is the women who have changed, not the men.

It is clear that there are profound physical, psychological, interpersonal, biological and social factors influencing a relationship following the birth of a child. On the one hand, pregnancy brings many couples closer together, with increased sharing in the great joy of bringing up a child together. On the other hand, it is clear that becoming a parent brings anxieties and tensions and the need to change and adapt (Box 9.2).

SEXUALITY IN THE MIDDLE AND LATER YEARS

Menopause

Changes associated with the menopause are discussed in Chapter 8. In this chapter we focus specifically on sexuality at that time. After the menopause, women are perfectly able to maintain interest and pleasure in sex, and for some this may be enhanced because the fear of pregnancy is over and periods have stopped.

Women's responses to the menopause are, to a large extent, shaped by their previous psychosexual relationships; their attitudes towards themselves and their sexuality; and their current situation and career/work commitment. For those with high self-esteem, in a happy partnership, enjoying a satisfying sexual relationship, the menopause usually constitutes a relatively easy transition. For others, who have never enjoyed sexual intercourse, and have viewed it as a 'chore' or a 'duty', there may be a sense of relief since they can use the menopause as an excuse not to have sex. However, even when women have previously enjoyed their sexual lives, there may be a feeling that after the menopause it is no longer 'proper' to enjoy sex. For some, sexual satisfaction is bound up with procreation, and it may be difficult to feel a sexual person when fertility ceases.

Several circumstances may make the menopause a more difficult transition. When there have been previous losses such as miscarriage, ectopic pregnancy or termination of pregnancy, the end of fertility may provoke past distress and sadness about these events, particularly if a child was very much wanted but never achieved. There may be feelings of grief and mourning at the menopause for infertile couples or single women who have struggled with infertility, undergoing medical and surgical treatments but never conceiving a child. For them the menopause marks the final closing of the door, sometimes leading to a sense of futility, failure and emptiness. Sexuality at the menopause may also be more fraught if the partner is 'youth-orientated'. Some men feel that remaining youthful is tied up with their sexuality in a way that makes them seek younger women.

An unusually early menopause can sometimes bring overwhelming feelings of ceasing to be a sexual person. A 25-year-old woman going through the menopause described her feelings in terms of many losses:

> *Part of me and my life has gone. A lot of the best parts – my fertility, my youth, my future being a mum and a grandma. I'm left with feeling old and my body doesn't work properly. I've got to take HRT now – just like my mum and all her friends. The worst thing is what's my husband going to think of me now, married to this sort of woman.*

Older ages

In our society, the over-65s are now a fast-growing proportion of the population, with many leading healthy, independent lives and enjoying their sexuality. Living an active, fulfilling life is, to a large extent, helped (but not guaranteed) by the maintenance of good health.

On the whole, in later life, the frequency of sexual intercourse falls, but this depends on:

◆ patterns of intercourse from earlier years
◆ general interest in sex
◆ availability of an interested partner
◆ degree of privacy
◆ general and local health considerations.

Both partners need to understand the physical aspects of the ageing process that are likely to affect intercourse:

- reduced swelling of the clitoris and labia during intercourse may decrease sensation
- reduced vaginal lubrication may increase the risk of painful sex
- loss of local muscle tone may reduce sensation for both partners
- sexual arousal is likely to take longer.

Despite these changes, most older women and men continue to enjoy sex albeit less frenetically than when younger. Sexuality is not confined to orgasm; it includes caressing, expressions of affection and intimacy.

Rising divorce rates (as well as bereavement) mean many women are starting new sexual relationships, sometimes after years of celibacy. For them the upsurge in sexual activity may not only be pleasurable but may also bring anxieties.

On the whole, men find it more difficult than women to express fears about their sexuality and often present to their doctor with more 'respectable' symptoms, or add a concern as if it were an afterthought. As Mr Jones gets up from his chair in the doctor's consulting room, he says hesitantly, with his hand on the door, 'Oh, there is just one more thing I forgot to mention, doctor.' Sometimes the anxiety is about ageing; or about failing to please his partner, or there may be anger and resentment of expectations that differ from those of his partner. Ageing is a mental and physical transition, much influenced by social context and with strong implications for couple interactions and sexuality.

Case study 9.2

Mrs Jones, aged 67, attended the well woman clinic asking for a check-up. When I asked her what sort of check-up she was hoping for she appeared uncertain and anxious. 'I'm too old for a smear test, aren't I, but I just wondered if you could see if I'm alright there?'

I asked her if she felt something was wrong. 'Well, I'm not sure. I'm a bit worried – I haven't had sex for over 10 years now since I lost my first husband and I'm just going to get married again. I feel a bit scared about starting sex again. I've no idea what my vagina's like now. I've never taken HRT and I wonder if it's all dried up?' She was relieved when I said we could do a vaginal examination together. She agreed I would examine her first and then she said she would like to feel herself. She was relaxed and easy to examine, and her vagina and pelvic floor felt normal with reasonable muscle tone. She was relieved to hear this and agreed that she would examine herself with me close at hand. This she did and to her surprise said, 'I never thought it would be so easy and normal – I think I'm alright aren't I?'

We continued to talk about her plans for her new life, and she showed her excitement and happiness. It appeared she was in touch again with her vagina and the prospect of her renewed sexuality.

Some older women are most likely to find intimacy in remarriage, especially if they view sex as only possible within a married relationship. However, opposition may come from children and grandchildren. Older children may feel critical and resentful of the sexuality of their parent and may feel they are behaving in a 'ridiculous' way. This can be particularly so when there is an older woman/younger man relationship. In this case, it may be that the children have never come to terms with their mother's sexuality.

CONCLUSION

Sexuality has many dimensions and impinges on, and is affected by, many different psychological and physical features. However, more than anything else, it concerns social relationships. In the next chapter, their development is discussed with respect to the life span course and its implications for practice.

BIBLIOGRAPHY

Montford H, Skrine R (eds) 1987 Contraceptive care. Chapman & Hall, London
This book focuses on the body/mind approach to contraception demonstrating the insights and skills needed by practitioners with the use of extensive case histories.

Skrine R 1997 Blocks and freedoms in sexual life. Radcliffe, Oxford
This book uses case histories to explore skills used in understanding human sexuality and the relationships between the body and the mind. The focus of the study is on the doctor/patient relationship and what happens between two people in an encounter as well as observing what is going on in the physical examination.

REFERENCES

Ashmore R D, DelBoca F K, Wohlers A J 1986 Gender stereotypes. In: Ashmore R D, DelBoca F K (eds) The social psychology of female–male relations: a critical analysis of central concepts. Academic Press, New York, pp 69–119
Bancroft J 1989 Human sexuality and its problems, 2nd edn. Churchill Livingstone, Edinburgh
Bozett F 1981 Gay parents. Alternative Lifestyles 4: 90–108
Fishbein M, Ajzen I 1972 Attitudes and opinions. Annual Review of Psychology 23: 487–544
Golombok S, Fivush R 1994 Gender development. Cambridge University Press, Cambridge
Gorski R A 1996 Gonadal hormones and the organization of brain structure and function. In: Magnusson D (ed) The lifespan development of individuals. Cambridge University Press, Cambridge, pp 315–340
Hofferth S L, Hayes C D (eds) 1987 Risking the future: adolescent sexuality, pregnancy and childbearing. 2. Working papers and statistical appendixes. National Academy Press, Washington, DC
Hogan R 1980 Human sexuality: a nursing perspective. Appleton-Century-Crofts, New York

Langlois J H, Downs A C 1980 Mothers, fathers and peers as socialization agents of sex-typed play behaviours in young children. Child Development 51: 1237–1247

Lees S 1986 Losing out: sexuality and adolescent girls. Hutchinson Education, London

Maccoby E E, Jacklin C N 1980 Sex differences in aggression: a rejoinder and reprise. Child Development 51: 964–980

Moore S, Rosenthal D 1992 Sexuality in adolescence. Routledge, London

Moss P, Bolland G, Foxman R, Owen C 1986 Marital relations during the transition to parenthood. Journal of Reproductive and Infant Psychology 4: 57–67

Orbach S 1991 What is going on here? Virago, London

Pawlby S J, Mills A, Quinton D 1997a Vulnerable adolescent girls. Opposite sex relationships. Journal of Child Psychology and Psychiatry 38: 909–920

Pawlby S J, Mills A, Taylor A, Quinton D 1997b Adolescent friendships mediating childhood adversity and adult outcomes. Journal of Adolescence 20: 633–644

Raphael-Leff J 1991 Pregnancy: the inside story. Sheldon Press, London

Robson K M, Brant H A, Kumar R 1981 Maternal sexuality during first pregnancy and after childbirth. British Journal of Obstetrics and Gynaecology 88: 9

Rutter M 1980 Psychosexual development. In: Rutter M (ed) Scientific foundations of developmental psychiatry. William Heinemann, London

Rutter M, Rutter M 1993 Developing minds: challenge and continuity across the life span. Penguin, London

Rutter M, Giller H, Hagell A 1998 Antisocial behaviour by young people. Cambridge University Press, Cambridge

Savin-Williams R C 1994 Gay and lesbian youth. Expressions of identity. Hemisphere, Washington, DC

Southern M 1994 Labour and sexuality. Midwifery Matters 61: 5

Taylor V J 1992 Pregnancy: a shared experience? Men's experiences and feelings about their partner's pregnancy. Journal of Advances in Health and Nursing Care 2:2–59

Van Wert W F 1991 Sex after childbirth. Mothering 60:115

Wellings K, Field J, Johnson A M, Wadsworth J 1994 Sexual behaviour in Britain. Penguin, London

10

The growth of social relationships

Marjorie Rutter

KEY ISSUES

◆ Relationships as an important part of development
◆ The qualities of attachment relationships and the importance of attachments
◆ Different patterns of attachment
◆ Loss of relationships including divorce and re-marriage
◆ The nature of social relationships
◆ Peer relationships and emotional problems

INTRODUCTION

The capacity to form intimate social relationships is a fundamental part of human nature. Much of what people learn throughout the course of their lives comes about in the context of relationships. That is so with respect to language and communication; it is so for many facets of sexuality; and it applies equally in the field of emotions. The stress of broken relationships, personal rebuffs and rejection, and entrapment in a conflictual partnership constitutes a prime precipitant of emotional disturbance. Similarly, the protective effect of a close warm supportive relationship provides a crucial buffering role in enabling people to cope with life challenges and adversity.

Social development begins in infancy and continues throughout life as individuals face new social demands, opportunities and problems. This chapter considers how this comes about and discusses the implications for clinical practice. Even newborn babies exhibit social qualities but during the first year these undergo dramatic transformations as selective attachments to caregivers emerge and come to occupy an increasingly important role in many other aspects of behaviour, emotional adjustment and social competence.

This chapter explores the qualities of selective attachments and the ways in which they may lead on to, and shape other types of relationships such as friendships with peers, romances, sexual relationships and parenting of their own children. As individuals experience interactions and relationship with other people, they develop an understanding of themselves and of others' responses to them in social encounters. That understanding, or self-concept, will in turn influence how they deal with later relationships.

Children, as they grow older, become better able to maintain relationships during a period of separation but the experience of a loss of an important relationship remains a stressor throughout life. Such losses are discussed in terms of the ways in which they impinge at different ages, and of the fact that susceptibilities tend to be increased at the time of adversity or illness.

One of the key features of development is that people differ in their patterns. One aspect of such individuality concerns the differences between males and females in their approach to relationships and another concerns the extent to which people feel secure in their relationships and in the role of sexuality in such relationships. These differences matter for clinical practice.

RELATIONSHIPS AS AN IMPORTANT PART OF DEVELOPMENT

Beginnings of social relationships

Children are born into a complex social world and from the first weeks of life they are active participants in interactions with other people (Dunn 1988). These interactions influence the development of cognition, language, emotion and social behaviour. Their quality will depend not only on the personality of the child and the carers but also on the structures, norms and expectations of the groups that make up the child's social world.

The child seeks to understand the intentions, feelings and actions of others and to make sense of the rules of that environment. Babies are born predisposed to learn about sights and sounds of the people around them. Infants of 2–3 months develop the ability to perceive actions and expressions of other people (Stern 1985). For example, they are least likely to respond when presented with an expressionless face and most likely to do so when mother or father laughs and talks in a responsive way. There is an increasing sociability during the first 6 months and interchanges with the baby are like a dialogue with parents timing their responses to fit in with baby's smiles and vocalisations. Babies often initiate 'conversations' by making their own noises to attract the attention of their parents, or practise new sounds to enlarge their repertoire. Infants are most responsive to sounds of the human voice. As a result of these interactions they develop their powers of communication, understanding and thought, their emotional security and sense of themselves. This sense of self and being in control develops initially through control of objects, toys, their own limbs and voice. Gradually, attempts are made to control the actions of others by laughing, crying, screaming and smiling, and later on by pointing and gesturing.

Babies are tuned into different emotional expressions of the mother and respond differently and appropriately to these expressions. If they observe their mothers interacting positively with a stranger they are less wary of that stranger subsequently than babies whose mothers interact neutrally (Feiring et al 1984). Being a social person, whether infant or adult, involves trying to discover what others are thinking and feeling. By 9 months babies are beginning to join in games such as peek-a-boo with others and are able to cooperate in feeding themselves. These achievements indicate the child's ability to take control and begin to make decisions about their lives and show the beginnings of separation from the caregiver.

The qualities of attachment relationships

Selective attachment relationships begin to form from about 6 months of age (but have their antecedents in much earlier social interchanges), and the quality of these relationships influences social and emotional development. Children may have several selective attachments, which are likely to include siblings and other family members. However, there is a marked hierarchy with the mother, as the primary caregiver, usually at the top because she has been the person most available to reduce anxiety at key moments. The quality of the attachment relationship is important to the degree that it provides the child with:

◆ Security, when she is frightened, upset, tired, ill or in a strange situation.
◆ A secure base, from which she can explore her surroundings. Initially, children stay close to their mother but gradually they make forays further afield returning at intervals for reassurance, comfort, or emotional and physical nourishment.
◆ Protection against stress.
◆ Continuity of care, so that the prime caregiver is consistently a valuable source of support.
◆ Sensitivity and warmth in response to needs within an intimate relationship.

The importance of attachments

It seems that these qualities enable the child to feel comfortable with closeness and confident that others will be helpful. A secure attachment relationship is likely to foster:

◆ self-reliance
◆ competence with peers
◆ sociable relationships with adults
◆ empathy and help for others in distress.

Attachments develop, even in the face of maltreatment and severe punishment. Indeed most young children or young animals are most likely to cling when frightened or upset. If no one else is available they will cling to the person who is maltreating them (Bowlby 1969). Not all children have the experience of a secure attachment during this period and, as we have noted in the case study of Samantha in Chapter 8, her early experiences had shaping effects on her life. However, the course of development is not fixed and, therefore, when people have subsequent good experiences at school or in work situations, as well as a sensitive, supportive relationship, development may be shifted on to a more favourable path. There is a continuing potential for change, as Helen's story (p. 175) highlights.

Different patterns of attachment insecurity

Attachment theory and findings have been important for years in translating the rather diffuse concept of 'mother love' into specific biologically based aspects of parent–child interactions and relationships, and in emphasising that this was not the whole of parenting (Bowlby 1969). Thus, mother love functions differently from play and from discipline. Ainsworth's (1967) research was also crucial in the demonstration of the importance of differentiating secure and insecure attachment qualities and in providing a brief observational method – the 'Strange Situation' (based on very short periods of separation and reunion) – to measure them (Ainsworth et al 1978). She highlighted two main types of insecure attachment – 'anxious-avoidant' and 'anxious-resistant' – and one type of secure attachment. All these are normal in the sense that they are common in the general population (about a third to a half of children are rated as having an insecure relationship). However, secure attachments are ordinarily more adaptive in that the attachment relationship enables the child to feel safe and to have confidence to be apart from the caregiver when older.

At first, the secure/insecure qualities apply to just one specific relationship but gradually, over time, the experiences of that relationship, and other attachment relationships, over multiple circumstances, provide the child with what has come to be called an 'internal working model' of relationships. In other

Case study 10.1

Helen came to a clinic after trying for a baby for 2 years. She was now 43 years old and over the age limit for treatment. Helen had experienced a wide range of distressing experiences as a child, beginning with her father's abandonment of the family when she was 2 years old. Her mother became depressed and reliant on Helen for comfort and solace and they began to sleep together. However, when Helen started school her mother began a relationship with a man who very soon moved into the home and quickly took Helen's place in mother's bed. He had no time for Helen, who felt rejected by her mother's attention to the new boyfriend whom she very quickly married. Helen began to have nightmares, fear of the dark and bedwetting for which she was punished. She often truanted from school. At 16 she became pregnant and her stepfather attempted to beat her up. She ran away from home to stay with her aunt, Margaret, who supported her through the termination of pregnancy and took care of her. They developed a close and trusting relationship and Margaret helped Helen get a job at the local GP surgery. She had a few boyfriends over the next few years but found it difficult to have a close sexual relationship. Unfortunately, Margaret died very suddenly of a heart attack and Helen was devastated at the loss and at being alone again. However, she continued her work at the surgery, which provided her with support, friendship and stability. She became interested in aromatherapy and trained to become a practitioner. She started work in an Alternative Medicine Centre where she met John, who was 39. They fell in love and for the first time Helen felt she could trust a man with her feelings. They began to try for a child but were unsuccessful for 2 years and also failed after 18 months of assisted conception. When Helen came she said, 'I'm not sure why I'm here – I just know I've got to end all this – I'm too old. I thought I'd never get over not having a baby, it's all I wanted at one time – someone to love me and me to love them. But I've changed now. I've got John and he's changed my life. I'm so happy. I think I've done very well.'

words, the child comes to have a general expectation that close relationships will be secure or insecure and, in this way, develops a self-concept and a concept of others that goes beyond a single relationship (see section below on cognitive sets).

The secure/insecure classification was based on studies of children reared in relatively ordinary circumstances. It became clear later that this did not necessarily pick out the key unusual features in children whose upbringing was markedly different (as, for example, because of an institutional rearing or the experience of chronic abuse or gross parental psychopathology). Also, it was not entirely satisfactory when insecure features formed part of a broader pattern of maladaptation. The category of 'disorganised attachment' was introduced to deal with this need (Main and Solomon 1990).

Children whose early attachment relationships lack security tend to be more likely to have difficulties in later loving, intimate relationships. These include:

◆ undue jealousy in close relationships
◆ feelings of loneliness even when involved in a relationship
◆ reluctance to commitment in relationships
◆ a tendency to view partners as insufficiently attentive (see Robert's story in Chapter 3, pp 56–57).

It is also apparent that some adults who experienced poor parenting when young tend to be less able to provide sensitive caregiving for their own children. Clinical evidence suggests that a mother's feelings and behaviour towards her child are influenced by the experiences she had, and may still be having, with her own parents. Comforting others in distress is a pattern that frequently develops in the second year of life and this is influenced by how parents treat their child (Ellis 1982). However, many people who have experienced a stressed upbringing become excellent parents. It may be important for people to accept the reality of their own poor parenting and understand and use the important qualities of subsequent good relationships to allow them to have a positive view of themselves as good parents.

Early attachments and the shaping of later relationships

Selective attachments reflect the importance of both continuity and sensitive responsiveness in caregiving as features of a child's upbringing (Rutter & O'Connor 1999). The presence of selective attachments in the first 3 or 4 years of life are particularly influential because they come first and because they provide such a crucial experience of intimacy. Pincus (1997) described marriage as providing the lost world of earlier intimacy where he 'enjoyed the physical gratification of another's body, commanded paramount loyalty and was in fact the centre of that other person's life'. It seems that the qualities of early attachment relationships play a role in shaping later relationships – friendships with peers, love relationships, parental relationships with one's own children and sexual relationships (Rutter 1995). The relationships created are dynamic, each influencing the other and in turn being influenced by other past and current relationships. As practitioners, we are aware that some of these qualities are of great value in professional roles. For example, whether in practice or supervision our work relies on the qualities of warmth and generosity for emotional support and reduction of anxiety (Faugier 1992). An individual's experience of one sort of relationship tends to shape their experience of and approach to later relationships.

Selective attachments do not just apply to infants; they also concern aspects of relationships that reduce anxiety and provide emotional protection and comfort in times of stress. It is evident that these qualities apply across the life span into extreme old age. Of course, attachment qualities constitute just one feature of relationships, however important, and the experiences of play, conversations, discipline and supervision are also influential. Intense relationships between parents and children, siblings, lovers and close friends all tend to have an exclusive quality and when this exclusiveness is threatened by the other person's relationships with another, feelings of rivalry and jealousy may arise. For example, all children need to feel valued by their parents and when siblings are born they may begin to feel less well treated or not so favoured; feelings that may persist into adult life. Sibling relationships show surprising continuity over time (Dunn & Kendrick 1982). The desire for close relationships is an important part of being human and if one relationship is failing, compensation may be sought in another one. Mothers who are in an unhappy marital relationship or whose partner has abandoned the family, may develop an overprotective and dependent relationship with one of their children (see case study of Helen earlier in this chapter).

Separations

Once specific attachments have been formed, children tend to protest at being separated from their mother or primary caregiver. This protest is most marked in the toddler period; it then wanes gradually as children gain the ability to maintain images of people during periods of absence and hence learn to keep relationships over times of separation.

As children get older they venture steadily further from their base for increasing spans of time. They come to gain an increasing sense of security without the need for the parent to be physically close. They become able to understand the reasons for parents being away for short periods and they learn to accept comfort from others.

For most people, separations throughout life can be clearly evoked – first day at school, leaving home for the first time, saying goodbye to a good friend. Feelings of sadness, loss and anxiety about coping when an important source of support and care is gone, are all experiences of separation. For most people, they can be managed without too much distress because there will usually be other supportive people around. However, when separations coincide with other stressful life events, such as illness, then people may become particularly vulnerable.

LOSS OF RELATIONSHIPS (see also Chapter 5)

Loss of a loved one

The grieving process is influenced by the quality of the lost relationship, and especially by its attachment features. The loss of a loved one may bring up fear and panic of being left alone with no-one to turn to, lack of support, comfort and security, and feelings of abandonment (Pincus 1997).

Grief reactions are intensely personal and each person negotiates mourning in a different way. Sometimes people feel so overwhelmed and vulnerable that they build defences against their neediness and their feelings of loneliness and grief. Others may feel that, after a certain length of time, expressions of grief are unacceptable (Box 10.1).

Parkes & Markus (1998) have documented the course of grief in adults:

◆ **Numbness** – difficulty realising that the death has happened.
◆ **Pain** of the loss – longings for the dead person that may involve thoughts of having seen or heard them
◆ **Restlessness** and **agitation** – sometimes leading to a frenzy of activity
◆ **Difficulty sleeping**
◆ **Anger** – directed towards the dead person, family members, or to the doctors who 'let it happen'
◆ **Comfort-seeking** and **comfort rejecting**.

Pain and distress may go on for many months or years and may involve despair and depression. As the pain recedes, life usually becomes re-established but the pain may resurface at times of anniversaries.

Hidden losses

Death and loss are sometimes surrounded by secrecy and taboo. Thus, many patients fail to tell their practitioners about early miscarriages, ectopic or terminated pregnancies. These are often hidden losses, sometimes kept secret,

---

Box 10.1 Features associated with very disturbed grief reactions

◆ an ambivalent or unduly dependent relationship with the person who died, so that negative and positive feelings complicate the grieving process
◆ an unexpected or untimely death, as with the death of a child
◆ the coincidence of death with other stresses or life crises such as a family row or loss of a job
◆ previous losses that have been incompletely resolved.

Features associated with less disturbing grief reactions:

◆ the availability and effective use of social supports from friends and family
◆ the re-establishment of life patterns
◆ the development of new intimate relationships
◆ the provision of crisis intervention.

sometimes never mourned, but which can give rise to overwhelming feelings of vulnerability (see case study below).

Case study 10.2

A couple had been trying unsuccessfully for a child for 5 years when they finally accepted that they were unable to create a child. They talked of their feelings of emptiness and hopelessness but felt very alone, finding it difficult to grieve. There was no 'real' child to mourn, only the hope and longing for one who was acutely real but never existed.

Grief may interfere with sexual responsiveness and couples may feel that sex is inappropriate in sorrow. However, for some couples, sex is an important way of giving and receiving comfort.

Grief reactions in children

It is apparent that children do grieve but, on the whole, their immediate grief reactions are less intense and prolonged than in adults. Probably this is because children tend not to project their thinking forwards and backwards in the same way as do adults. The young tend to be less inclined to dwell on the failings of the past or their fears for the future. However, children need to be able to talk about death and what has happened, so that they can make sense of it in their own way. Sometimes grief is made more difficult because children have been 'protected' from the rituals and rites of bereavement, with the result that their grief is not acknowledged and shared. Bereaved siblings need to feel accepted, to have their fears allayed that death is unlikely to spirit them away and that their own irrational, but very real, sense of blame is unfounded. Helping children through their grief may provide grieving parents with an outlet and solace for their own sense of loss (Raphael-Leff 1993).

The situation may be different and more complex for children when a parent dies, and the children may have to:

1. cope with the grief of the surviving parent as well as their own grief
2. try to survive the possible adverse effects on the quality of parental care, which may be associated with depression
3. experience irrational fears and fantasies that in some way they may have contributed to the death.

Parental divorce

Loss is an important element in a child's or young person's reaction to parents splitting up, but the distress and disturbance is also frequently due to previous parental conflict and disturbed family relationships. However, children may become upset by feelings of guilt, thinking that they caused the break-up. They may strive to find ways of bringing their parents together again. Childrens' problems following divorce are more likely to arise if there is continuing discord and conflict and if the custodial parent becomes depressed. As in other stressful situations, where there are other close caring supports, e.g. grandparents, there is more likely to be a better adaptation.

Parental remarriage

Hetherington (1989) followed up children of divorced parents over a 6-year period and examined their reactions to remarriage; results are shown in Box 10.2.

Hetherington found that girls who had a warm, close relationship with their mother *before* remarriage were more likely to have a conflicted one afterwards – a feeling of loss of a special relationship rather than any gain (see Helen's story earlier in this chapter). In Chapter 11 the effects of divorce on adults are considered.

THE NATURE OF SOCIAL UNDERSTANDING

Understanding others' feelings and social rules

During the second and third years of life children begin to understand the connection between their own actions and another person's state of pain, anger or amusement, and their powers of understanding are often used in struggles to gain their own way (Dunn 1988). A child develops an understanding of others' intentions and feelings through the dynamic interactions with their own family and friends. Their experiences of punishment, kindness and sharing are all understood through these important relationships.

Box 10.2 Reactions to remarriage

Mother:
1. Her mental state improves.
2. There is a marked improvement in economic and living conditions of mother and child(ren).

Child:
1. Boys tend to benefit more than girls.
2. Younger children are more likely to benefit, whereas adolescents are less likely to accept a new parental relationship.

Children also begin to understand social rules. They refer to sharing and taking turns when in competition with their sibling, but the rules may be used in an indirect way to 'get at' the sibling. Rules of possession also become understood with the increasing use of possessive pronouns, i.e. 'that's mine'.

Children become more aware that other people have feelings and intentions different from their own, e.g. their mother's moods, their sibling's intentions. They become sensitive to the responses of others in the form of support, approval and disapproval. Emotions encountered in these interactions, like anger on distress, may make them more attentive to others' behaviour, so that they remember, reflect on and learn from the impact of those encounters. The emotional content of an experience profoundly affects the way in which it is remembered and hence how it affects functioning.

Cognition and cognitive sets

Childrens' cognitive development takes place within their social world and is influenced by other people. Children use other people's knowledge in their own development, and the ways in which other people treat them shape their own understanding about themselves and others. We are influenced by people's reputation, gender and social standing as well as by our overall view of the situation. If an experience is viewed as negative then it is more likely to leave feelings of inadequacy, self- blame, helplessness and low self-esteem.

From their experiences people develop a set of 'cognitions' about them-selves, their relationships and their interactions with their environment. These cognitive sets are typically multifaceted. Thus, we may have a positive view of ourselves in relation to our work but feel inadequate in our friendships. We may feel generally good about ourselves (high self-esteem), yet lack confidence in our ability to deal with new challenges (low self-efficacy). These self-concepts tend to be persistent and are influential in how we deal with new relationships and new stresses. Equally, however, they are open to change if new experiences provide a different picture of success and failure.

Hammen's (1990) study illustrated the negative effects for children of depressed mothers – persistent maternal criticism led to both low self-esteem and low self-efficacy in dealing with stress. On the other hand, Pedersen et al's (1978) study of an outstanding primary school teacher illustrated positive effects. The teacher had a major, immediate direct effect on children's academic achievement and more substantial indirect effects over the longer term, i.e. children acquired styles of work and behaviour that brought success, which in turn reinforced their efforts. Possibly, too, their behaviour in class made them more rewarding pupils for teachers of later classes, who then responded to them in ways that facilitated success.

Understanding others' minds

During their third year children begin to talk about knowing, remembering and forgetting – both in themselves and others. There is an increasing curiosity about others, which is reflected in their stories. Language becomes more complex and is used in appropriate ways for making requests, responding to invitations and generally knowing how to master the situation and take control.

There are substantial individual differences in children's propensity to show empathy and in their tendency to exhibit prosocial behaviour; both remain moderately stable over time. Factors influencing these differences are:

1. The way in which they themselves have been treated.
2. Those children whose parents talk about other children's feelings and reactions are more likely to show comforting behaviour to others.
3. Abused children tend to respond aggressively to other people's distress.
4. Children exposed to family conflict, but not abused, tend to respond more than other children to adults' angry behaviour, and tend to show distress and concern. Toddlers respond to background anger.

Children tend to be upset when parents quarrel in front of them. It is apparent that some adults with this earlier experience continue to feel distress in the face of angry behaviour, and find this emotion very frightening and difficult to manage. In general, children of an unhappy relationship are likely to be aware of some underlying anger or distance between their parents. Perhaps they no longer kiss, eat, or sleep together. The parents may have little energy and be too preoccupied with their own unhappiness to attend to the child's needs, which may give rise to the child feeling isolated. However, a child may be able to find support, approval and recognition outside the home from teachers at school or other family members, such as grandparents. Children most at risk in the conflict are those who are 'put in the middle' through being used by one or both parents as allies or messengers (Parkes & Markus 1998).

Pre-school children are able to talk about mixed feelings but it takes longer for them to gain insight into their own emotional lives and to be aware of ambivalent emotions. By the age of about 6 they are able to hide emotions and are beginning to understand how this can be protective in certain circumstances. At this time children are also learning to control and regulate their emotions. Younger children tend to switch situations so that they experience something more enjoyable in order to counter distress; older children realise that painful feelings may prevent concentration but also that concentration can block out painful feelings. In clinical practice we see people who use this strategy of concentration to avoid emotional pain, and there is also an awareness that when people are miserable, not only do they tend to focus on negative experiences, but they are more likely to recall negative ones than happy ones.

Peer relationships and gender segregation

It is striking that from the pre-school years onwards, children tend to prefer playing with children of the same sex. The tendency to form sex-segregated groups increases in middle childhood, but is evident by the age of 3 when children are left to their own devices, unsupervised by adults. Different childhood 'cultures' prevail in these gender-segregated groups and sex segregation seems to be largely brought about by children's concepts of themselves as boys or girls. The drift into these groups is also found in non-industrial and non-Western societies. Boys and girls can interact effectively when situations are structured by teachers and adults, but this does not alter their underlying preference (Maccoby 1998).

Differences in boys' and girls' play styles

Boys' play styles

Boys tend to be more physical in their play than girls and this tends to take place in larger groups, with the focus around issues of dominance and the formation of a pecking order. They are more combative than girls in their verbal interactions, and use threats, boasts and joke-telling as a means of establishing power. They often enact warlike games using the roles of soldiers, policemen or cowboys. This competition is not normally aggressive, and often there is much cooperation within a group in order to beat the other group. Competition and cooperation are woven into their social relationships. Boys usually take more interest than girls in sport, watch more sport on TV, and talk more often about sport and sporting figures.

Girls' play styles

Girls tend to play in clusters of two or three and there is a strong convention of turn-taking. Girls tend to exert influence over others by complimenting other girls, requesting advice, asking favours or imitating. They tend to have difficulty dealing with conflict and, when it occurs, girls more often retaliate by manipulating the other girls' friendships. Girls' play frequently involves cooperative role-taking, e.g. 'you be the teacher' or 'you be the child', with family or school scenarios the most frequent. Their play-acting may include the preparing and serving of food, looking after guests, nurturing activities such as feeding and comforting the baby and using dolls. They may also act out scenarios of glamour and romance using dressing-up clothes such as bridal dresses and ball gowns. Girls are more likely to disclose their feelings, including their weaknesses, and share emotions as a way of maintaining positive relationships (Maccoby 1998).

Children begin to talk much more in their play from the age of 3, and at first boys and girls talk to their same-sex playmates in a similar manner, and then gradually begin to diverge and become more dissimilar by middle childhood. Girls' speech to each other tends to be more cooperative, reciprocal and collaborative. They also tend to have longer exchanges than boys and take turns and refer to themselves jointly. For example, 'We'll do …', or 'Why don't we …'. Girls do have disputes and confrontations but, on the whole, while pursuing their own objective they negotiate with others and consider others' wishes. Boys are more likely to pursue their own objectives and less likely to consider other peoples' wishes. They tend to use more domineering phrases such as 'give me' or 'put it there'.

Cross-gender encounters

The two different cultures of childhood are not totally disconnected. Most children are in close contact with the opposite sex at home, with siblings, family friends, or playmates down the road. Boys and girls are very much aware of each other and interactions usually start in groups where there is chasing and girls' teams competing against boys' teams. By age 9 or 10 the contacts are beginning to have romantic or sexual overtones. Love letters and invitations to meet secretly are common. Cross-sex teasing increases and dares to kiss and talk about dating and marrying become more frequent. Even at this early age there can be strong feelings of rejection and failure associated with these encounters.

Male and female interaction styles

It is interesting to follow these different interaction styles into adult life, although we need to appreciate that there are huge individual differences. Tannen (1991) described some ways in which typical talk among women is different from typical talk among men, which can lead to misunderstandings. In an office, for example, there are frequently same-sex groups in which women chat about hairstyles, clothes, domestic concerns and children. In the male same-sex groups the typical chat is often about cars, sports and technological subjects. Women have a more collaborative style of communication, which may have consequences for their career development. Tannen (1991) noted that women often fail to take credit for their achievements saying 'we' finished a successful piece of work, whereas a man would be more likely to say 'I' finished it. Different communication styles are also apparent in relation to confrontation issues. Women tend to soften critical messages, whilst men are much more direct, being less uncomfortable about delivering criticism. Here we can see carry-overs of those same-sex groupings of childhood.

Parents' interactional styles with their children

Starting early in childhood there is an important way in which parents talk differently to their sons and daughters, i.e. they talk more about feelings with girls than boys. Maccoby (1998) suggested that this may stem from language acquisition being earlier in girls, may reflect a girl's greater willingness to listen and talk about emotions, or it may seem too 'soft' for boys. It is known that fathers put more pressure on boys not to cry or show fear or weakness. Whatever the reason, talk of feelings with parents does occur more frequently in daughters and this helps them in being able to be aware of other people's feelings in later life.

Another important difference is that parents of both sexes play more roughly with young boys than girls and fathers in particular play these games much more with their sons. The style of these interactions at home emerge in single-sex playgroups a bit later on.

Peer relationships and emotional problems

Peer relationships are important for three different reasons:

1. They have a predictive value. Children who are isolated and rebuffed by others have an increased risk of having later psychosocial difficulties.

2. The peer group, as a social context, has an influence on current behaviour. It has an influence in its own right and exerts a force on the individuals within it. If the group, as a whole, is involved with drug-taking or early sexual behaviour, these behaviours may be fostered in other members of the group.

3. The peer group is likely to influence the choice of partner. Individuals make choices from the people around them and choose partners holding the same values and attitudes as the group. These attitudes may have either positive or negative influences.

However, not all children become deeply involved in groups and some stay on the periphery, finding it more difficult to belong.

In adult life, as well as in childhood, social relationships are affected by emotional state. For example, people who are depressed are more difficult to live with. Children often have difficulty expressing their sadness or anxieties, or they may not have anyone who recognises their distress, or may feel they have no-one to turn to. For example, when parents are arguing or in the process of breaking up, it can be frightening and worrying for a child to speak about their fears. There may be bullying at school or pressures from teachers about passing tests. Hetherington (1983) found that when children were distressed their play and interactions with other children were affected. Problems in peer relationships may be the origin of negative experiences that impact on self-concept to create the feeling 'I am an unlovable person'.

Poor peer relationships as a predictor of social problems

Peer rejection acts as a stressor and rejected children tend to be targets of others' aggression. Their lack of social success leaves them less able to join in social activities with their peers and they are more likely to feel isolated, unhappy and stigmatised. Because they are not part of social groups they tend to lack support and are therefore less buffered against other stresses. Their lack of social involvement makes them more likely to miss out on learning social skills and gives rise to low self-esteem. Problems may stem from the deviant behaviour associated with the rejection. Rejection and aggression are closely linked and the problems are greater when the two occur together.

Poor interpersonal relationships and antisocial behaviour both tend to generate life stressors which carry an increased risk for depression. Robins (1966) found that antisocial boys grew up to experience more rebuffs, rejections and broken love relationships in adult life than other men and lost their jobs more frequently.

CONCLUSIONS

The growth of social relationships constitutes a central aspect of development because relationships constitute a key feature in human functioning, and because they have such a major bearing on emotions, sexuality and people's responses to stress and challenge. As such, their strong relevance for clinical practice is obvious. Several aspects of social development are particularly note-worthy. Individual characteristics both reflect and influence social interactions and, hence, shape social groups. In turn, the context and ethos of those groups (as illustrated by gender features) helps shape individuals and adds meaning to their experiences. Their thought processes (as shown by cognitive sets and self-concepts) do the same. The early years are important in providing the basis for later relationships but, as discussed further in the next chapter, experiences in adolescence and adulthood may enhance or counter those early effects according to their content and context.

BIBLIOGRAPHY

Bowlby J 1988 A secure base. Routledge, London
Rutter M 1981 Maternal deprivation reassessed. Penguin, London

REFERENCES

Ainsworth M D 1967 Infancy in Uganda: infant care and growth of attachment. John's Hopkins Press, Baltimore
Ainsworth M D, Blehar M C, Waters E, Walls S 1978 Patterns of attachment. Erlbaum, Hillsdale, NJ

Bowlby J 1969 Attachment and loss: 1. Attachment. Hogarth Press, London

Dunn J 1988 Beginnings of social understanding. Blackwell, Oxford

Dunn J, Kendrick C 1982 Siblings. Grant McIntyre, London

Ellis P L 1982 Empathy: a factor in antisocial behaviour. Journal of Abnormal Psychology 10: 123–134

Faugier J 1992 The supervisory relationship: clinical supervision and mentorship in nursing. Stanley Thomas, London

Feiring C, Lewis M, Starr M D 1984 Indirect effects and infants' reaction to strangers. Developmental Psychology 20: 485–491

Hammen C 1990 Advances in clinical psychology 13. Plenum, New York

Hetherington E M 1983 Socialization, personality and social development. In: Mussen's handbook of child development. Wiley, New York, Vol 4

Hetherington E M 1989 Coping with family transitions: winners, losers, and survivors. Child Development 60(1): 1–14

Maccoby E E 1998 The two sexes. Harvard University Press, Harvard

Main M, Solomon J 1990 Procedures for identifying infants as disorganised/disorientated during the Ainsworth Strange Situation. In: Greenberg M, Cicchetti D, Cummings E M (eds) Attachment during the pre-school years: theory, research and intervention. University of Chicago Press, Chicago

Parkes C M, Markus A 1998 Coping with loss. BMJ Publications, London

Pedersen E, Faucher T A, Eaton W W 1978 A new perspective on the effects of first grade teachers on children's subsequent adult status. Harvard Education Review 48: 1–31

Pincus L 1997 Death in the family. Faber and Faber, London

Raphael-Leff J 1993 Pregnancy: the inside story. Sheldon Press, London

Robins L 1966 Deviant children grown up. Williams & Wilkins, Baltimore

Rutter M 1995 Clinical implications of attachment concepts: retrospect and prospect. Journal of Child Psychology and Psychiatry 36: 549–571

Rutter M, O'Connor T G 1999 Implications of attachment theory for child care policies. In: Cassidy J, Shaver P R (eds) Theory, research and clinical applications. Guilford Press, London, pp 823–844

Stern D 1985 The interpersonal world of the child. Basic Books, New York

Tannen D 1991 You just don't understand. Virago Press, London

11

Life experiences and transitions in adolescence and adulthood

Marjorie Rutter

KEY ISSUES

- ◆ Life span concepts
- ◆ Adolescence
- ◆ Adulthood
- ◆ Parenthood
- ◆ Mid-life experiences
- ◆ Older age

INTRODUCTION

Experiences can have a substantial impact, either positive or negative, on development, but there are major individual differences in response, in part related to how challenges have been dealt with in the past. It is uncommon for early and late experiences to be entirely independent of one another. One reason is that by their behaviour people shape their interactions with other people, thereby selecting particular social groups or circumstances. A second reason is that early experiences tend to determine later experiences, e.g. children who leave school at the first opportunity will lack the scholastic attainments that are required for many jobs, or a teenage pregnancy may precipitate an unhappy marriage. On the other hand, if new experiences open up fresh opportunities, they may constitute a positive turning point. Conversely, if adult circumstances shut down opportunities they may serve as a negative turning point. In certain circumstances, infertility may act in this way. In this chapter we consider how experiences in the post-childhood years may serve to enhance or impede adaptive functioning.

LIFE SPAN CONCEPTS

Erikson (1950, 1959) was influential in getting people to think of development in life span terms and to appreciate the importance of viewing personality growth in its social context. Both concepts have stood the test of time and continue to shape thinking about developmental issues (Hetherington et al 1988, Rutter & Rutter 1993, Elder 1998). The early writings, however, also portrayed development in terms of age-defined stages and specific social 'tasks', or crises (such as identity and intimacy). These views have had to be modified in the light of evidence that there is considerable individual variation in both the timing and sequence of these features and in the developmental paths followed. Accordingly, in this chapter, life experiences and transitions in the post-childhood years are discussed in relation to particular issues as they apply to individuals, rather than in terms of a predictable progression across predetermined stages.

ADOLESCENCE

As discussed in Chapter 8, puberty constitutes the most obvious marker of adolescence in terms of the marked alterations in physique, hormonal changes and the acquisition of secondary sexual characteristics. These are accompanied by sexual urges and by the first romantic relationships. In addition, adolescence is marked by changes in thought processes, social relationships and expectations, life experiences, and psychological difficulties, all of which may have implications for sexuality.

Changes in thought processes

During adolescence, young people develop an increased ability to conceptualise and consider the meaning of their experiences, and think about themselves as distinct individuals. They become more able to monitor their thinking for its consistency and logic – or lack of these qualities. They are more likely to contemplate the past with feelings of guilt or shame or embarrassment, and to anticipate the future with feelings of apprehension, hope and with a clearer articulation of goals and aspirations. It is a time when most young people come to experience a better defined sense of their identity and of their failings and limitations as well as their skills and capacities. Often this sense goes through a variety of changes as young people get to know themselves and develop a clearer vision of what they want to be. Typically it is a time of idealism, as well as assertions of autonomy and independence (which usually go along with worries of whether they can cope with what is entailed).

Social relationships and expectations

In the past, adolescence was often portrayed as a time of inner turmoil and of alienation from the family. These views were based on professionals' clinical contacts with a minority of youngsters seeking help for psychological problems. Studies of the general population have made it clear that neither turmoil nor alienation are universal. There are significant shifts in the relationships that adolescents have with their parents as they seek to establish their independence, but most continue to want parental guidance on major issues (even if they rebel and confront on issues of dress, hairstyle and curfew). On the other hand, teenagers do come to rely on their peers for emotional support and companionship, and they are likely to be much influenced by peer group mores and values. In addition, relationships with adults outside the family (such as teachers or youth club leaders) may come to be increasingly important.

The extent to which these changing social relationships and expectations lead to successful coping or difficulties will be influenced by parental qualities as well as by the characteristics of the individual adolescent (Noller & Callan 1991). On the whole, the transitions are most likely to be negotiated in an adaptive way when there is:

◆ a combination of family closeness and respect for the adolescent's individuality and need for autonomy
◆ openness and responsiveness to other's views
◆ parental democratic communication style whereby adolescents are encouraged to make their own decisions and plans, be assertive and adopt their own point of view.

Too much use of power and criticism by parents seems to have negative effects for both adolescents and the family as a whole. The young person may feel that there is a generalised complaining and criticism, leading to the feeling that 'nothing is right'. It is helpful if parents can be specific about what it is that they disapprove of so that the issue can be discussed in context and not spill over into general 'nagging' about everything.

New life experiences

The move from primary to secondary school is a major change for most children. It involves a new peer group, the loss of a secure base in a single classroom, the need to relate to many different teachers, and the shift from being a responsible senior to an immature junior. School exams, competitiveness in sports and the taking on of responsibility all bring challenges as well as rewards. The opportunities for success expand but so do the chances of failure! Social relationships involve the same mixture. Close friendships and romantic ties are very satisfying but rebuffs, rejections and broken love relationships are also the source of much unhappiness and loss of self-esteem. Compared with the past, much more decision-making is needed. Adolescents need to make up their minds whether to experiment with drugs, and how much sexual intimacy to allow.

Psychological difficulties

Although adolescence is a time when young people are outgrowing some of the difficulties of earlier childhood, it is also a time when new ones become much more common. Dieting and eating disorders become very prevalent in girls; depressive problems increase in frequency, especially in girls; and suicidal attempts become much more common. Alcohol/drug misuse and antisocial behaviour also reach a peak in both males and females. It would be a mistake to see these difficulties as the 'norm' for this age period. Most young people go through the teenage years without any serious psychological disorder. Nevertheless, lesser problems of these kinds affect most teenagers to some degree. The reason for these striking age trends in psychopathology are surprisingly poorly understood but it is evident that both biological influences and experiential factors play a part. The importance for clinical practice in the field of sexuality is that these psychological difficulties are likely to impinge greatly on young people's development of romantic relationships and on their coping with all that sexuality entails.

Romantic relationships

Many young adolescents develop romantic relationships where there is no explicit sex, although there may be fantasies about it happening in the future. The feeling of 'being in love' can give rise to a rosy glow involving unreal perceptions and expectations. Sometimes young people experience wide swings of emotion from rapture to despair and vice-versa with the beginnings and endings of relationships. Sometimes the elation of 'being in love' can lead to irrational judgements, which may lead to the risk of unprotected sex.

ADULTHOOD

Continuity and change

As we turn to a consideration of experiences and transitions in adult life we need to understand what is carried forward from childhood. Obviously, this includes the styles of thinking, social qualities and skills, interactional features, and patterns of behaviour that constitute the essence of individuality (see Chapter 7). In addition, however, people may bring with them vulnerabilities to stress brought about by adverse experiences when young, together with ways of viewing life challenges and of coping with them. By the time adult life is reached, most individuals will have developed a self-concept and a coherence of psychological functioning that is moderately stable over time. The stability reflects well established habits of behaviour and a consistency deriving from the ways in which people's styles of interaction shape and select the environments they experience. In this way, although the specifics of environments change from year to year, people's behaviour tends to bring about continuities in advantage and disadvantage (see Chapter 8). However, a degree of change is also common. Sometimes this comes about because people have deliberately acted in a particular way to change their circumstances and sometimes because of experiences over which they have little control. Sandra's case illustrates one way this may come about.

Case study 11.1

Sandra, a lively, bright and intelligent teenager, came to a clinic at the age of 18 requesting contraception. She said that she had just had a talk at school from a 'Family Planning lady' and this had prompted her to come. She said, 'It came at the right time for me, I don't intend to go the way of my sister.' Sandra came from a severely disrupted family with many problems. Her mother had been depressed for some time, her father was in prison for severe assault and her sister, aged 16, had just become pregnant. Her mother had told Sandra's sister to 'get out' and Sandra said, 'I need to get out too'. Sandra planned to go to university in the autumn and had an offer of a place dependent on her grades. She said that she worked with her boyfriend in the evenings at his home. He too was hoping to go to university and their teachers expected them to do well. Sandra had a thoughtful, positive cooperative manner and was keen to start the pill.

I didn't see Sandra again, until by chance, I happened to see her on the maternity ward where she had just been delivered of her first child at the age of 35. She had achieved the university degree she wanted and was launched on a successful career in journalism. Whilst at university, she broke up with the boyfriend she had had at 18 and for a period rather lost confidence in herself. There was a further crisis when her mother turned to her for help when she was beaten up by her husband soon after his release from prison. Sandra described how she felt that her experience in taking the decision not to repeat her family's problems had given her strength to deal with later difficulties, but that her pleasure in her job and the support of her husband had also been crucial in dealing with her initial failure to conceive in her early 30s. Clearly, Sandra's personal qualities had been instrumental in enabling her to make her own way in life but, equally, her good experiences in adult life did much to reinforce her early successes.

Work and unemployment

Moving into the world of work with the first job is a challenging experience, often seen as a 'rite of passage' in the transition to adulthood. Work varies in its meaning for people, being a source of satisfaction for some, boredom for others and stress for yet others. The importance of work does not just lie in the content of the job; often the social contacts it brings are a vital element. Unfortunately, for many young people, there are few opportunities for work and the transition is to unemployment, at least for a while. The lack of a job may give rise to anxiety and resentment as well as financial difficulties, and may also mean absence of a source of self-esteem.

Work may also involve conflicts. Career demands may mean long hours and emotional investment, leaving little time for leisure, friendships and family. Women face particular difficulties in work and family responsibilities, and many find it difficult to 'wind down' in the evening. Professional women wishing to have a career and raise a family often face enormous dilemmas about when to start a family. Fear that taking time off to have a baby will mean career penalties become accompanied by an awareness that the biological clock may be running down. In most societies, women are expected to bear the main burden of child care, even when both partners go out to work (Wortman et al 1991, Golombok & Fivush 1994). Unequal division of labour can give rise to feelings of resentment in the relationship, with a negative effect on sexual feelings.

There is abundant evidence that, in most societies, men not only tend to occupy higher status jobs, but get paid more for them than their female counterparts. Nevertheless, for many women, work gives them a sense of being in control of their lives, provides a source of satisfaction and achievement, and increases their self-esteem. It also brings contacts with interests outside the relationship they may have.

The experience of involuntary unemployment is often associated with a deterioration in mental health – job loss may mean financial strains but other consequences may be psychologically just as important (Box 11.1).

Box 11.1 Psychological consequences of job loss

◆ feelings of failure
◆ loss of life satisfaction
◆ loss of work friends
◆ loss of social status and self-esteem.

The strains are usually felt throughout the family.

Aye, and it's affecting us all at home. Not just the money, which is a
problem as well, it's a strain to be in the house with nothing to do.
Me and the wife are arguing more than usual and even the kids are tetchy.
I'm even smoking and drinking a bit too much, even when I can't afford it.
(Fagin 1998 p. 70).

A woman may have to carry the financial burden and manage on very little money, which can mean going without essentials for herself to give these to her family. Nevertheless, losing a satisfying job will be a very different experience from losing a boring and stressful one. What is lost is not the job but the satisfaction derived from it.

Marriage

There is a growing tendency in most Western cultures for young people to live together without marrying, sometimes having children without a clear decision to make a lifetime commitment. This pattern can work well, but there may be stresses for one partner when the couple differ in their degree of commitment. For others, it is a matter of drifting or of an impulsive step to escape from a stressful family situation. In their follow-up of institution-reared girls, Quinton & Rutter (1988) found that many lacked a belief that they could control their lives, and therefore tended not to exercise planning in relation to key decisions such as those involving work or marriage. All too often, the consequence was an unhappy marriage to a man with many problems, together with a teenage pregnancy and all the risks that this entails for both the relationship and the children (see the case study of Samantha in Chapter 9, p. 148).

Nevertheless, for many young adults, marriage provides an intimate and enduring relationship that is a source of support, as well as pleasure. Sometimes we hear of people being 'transformed' by marriage, but this is rarely so, not least because people tend to marry people like themselves. In this way social patterns and environments tend to remain the same. However, marriage can be a turning point if the partner is chosen from a different background, and when the relationship provides security and stability (see the case study of Helen in Chapter 10, p. 175).

However, there seem to be important sex differences in the effects of marriage. On balance, marriage tends to be psychologically protective for men, but this is less evident for women. Married men differ from the single and divorced in having somewhat better mental health. Divorced women also experience worse health but there is not the difference between single and married women that is found in men.

Any close relationship requires negotiation over roles, responsibilities and division of tasks. Cultures vary in the extent to which male and female roles are defined differently and there have been changes over time in expectations. Despite large increases in the proportion of women having work careers, they continue to carry the major responsibilities for child care, and to a lesser extent, for housework. As discussed in Chapter 10, men and women tend to differ somewhat in their styles of communication and this may lead to difficulties in negotiation. Sometimes the way intimacy is dealt with can be a source of resentment, jealousy or anger. Although there is a marked overlap between the sexes, on the whole women tend to be more at ease in sharing emotions and in discussing difficulties; many men prefer a practical approach to problems, shying away from talk about their feelings. Often, too, men feel they have to be the strong one, taking the stresses and strains 'like a man' (see Case study 11.2).

Case study 11.2

Joan and Alan came to the fertility clinic for help. Joan became distressed as she described the heavy weight of grief and sadness that she carried around all the time. She felt very much alone with the pain. When I asked Alan how he felt he said, 'You can't let it get you down, you have to keep going. I've got to be strong and positive for us both. What good would it do if I let go?' I said, 'What is there to let go?' After a while he said, 'Feeling stupid and pathetic, nobody knows what it is like when you can't have a baby.'

Issues that arouse strong feelings in both partners may be difficult to resolve when each has a different way of coping with emotions. Coping with anger may give rise to loss of sexual feelings. Conflict involves dealing with one's own negative feelings as well as those expressed by the partner. Some relationships may be collusive, where both partners project the parts of themselves they cannot accept onto the other person which are then a further source of resentment (Main 1986).

The stress from being in an unhappy marriage substantially increases the risk of developing depression but, equally, the presence of depression in one partner puts a substantial strain on the marriage.

Risk factors for marital breakdown

Marriages fail for diverse reasons, but several factors point to an increased risk of discord and breakdown:

1. Persistent antisocial behaviour in childhood, giving rise to problems with close harmonious relationships

2. A lack of harmonious family relationships in the upbringing of one or both partners
3. Recurrent mental disorder
4. Social disadvantage, poverty and poor housing conditions
5. Marriages brought about by an unwanted pregnancy
6. Teenage marriage.

Marital separation

Close, confiding relationships are emotionally protective at all ages and the breakdown of a love relationship (whether by separation or divorce) is an important stressor throughout the life span. However, stress does not derive from an event itself but rather from the processes that lead up to, and follow, the break. These include the trauma associated with hostility and unresolved conflict, the loss of self-esteem that is associated with rejection and the impact on other relationships. Friends may take sides, or sever the friendship altogether. When couples decide that they can no longer continue their relationship, both partners are likely to experience some form of separation distress, which may take the form of severe grief or may be accompanied by relief at the prospect of an end to the discord. Feelings may include intense anger as well as uncertainties about personal worth and acceptability (Parkes & Markus 1998).

PARENTHOOD

Becoming a parent

Until they become parents, few men or women realise the magnitude of the change brought about by having a child. Becoming responsible for the care of a baby who is totally dependent on others for survival is a transforming experience, quite apart from the demands during the day and the stress of disturbed nights. This new relationship has implications for the marital or cohabiting relationship, and many men fear that their relationship with their partner will assume a secondary position compared with the one the mother has with the child (Taylor 1992). Women, too, may be anxious about their ability to cope with mothering, or deal with their loss of status in giving up work or continue to feel a sexual person.

As we have seen, challenges and stressful situations accentuate pre-existing personal characteristics and interpersonal relationships, rather than changing them, and these have implications for a relationship (Box 11.2). It is important therefore to recognise what has gone before.

> **Box 11.2** Relationships particularly vulnerable during the transition to parenthood
>
> Relationships where:
> 1. the woman has experienced previous psychological difficulty
> 2. there is pre-existing marital disharmony
> 3. there is a markedly poor mother–daughter relationship
> 4. the woman is a teenager
> 5. there are career/parenthood tensions
> 6. there is lack of social support
> 7. there is a sharp contrast between the expectations and the realities of motherhood
> 8. the infant is handicapped or the neonatal period is marked by illness or medical interventions.

Single parenting

The single-parent family is becoming increasingly common and most of these are led by women. For some, it is by choice, for others it is the force of circumstances. The decision to mother alone may reflect a deep-seated wish to maintain independence, or it may derive from fears about committed relationships with men. Some women leave relationships because they realise that they are lesbian and want to give up the pretence of heterosexuality. As well as being a time of discovery for themselves, there can be major uncertainties over informing family and friends; children, in particular, may feel bewildered by their mother's homosexuality (see Chapter 9).

Single motherhood is difficult for a variety of practical and emotional reasons. When it is a considered choice with ample social, emotional and economic supports it can work well for both mother and child. On the other hand, the combination of being the sole source of income and the prime caregiver can bring huge demands and stresses. The very fact of being unable to share any of this work with a partner adds to the difficulties. Often, too, the mother has difficulties in coping with her sexuality and with her need for friendship, support and understanding within a loving relationship. Ambivalent feelings about a new commitment can be confusing and the woman may be particularly vulnerable to accidentally becoming pregnant when she meets someone who seems caring. Unfortunately some single mothers rush into new relationships that all too frequently turn out to be unloving or violent, like the one that led to their becoming a single parent. However, many mothers come through an exceedingly demanding transition and say they would never go back to the former relationship. This is reflected in divorce figures, which show that twice as many women as men file for divorce.

Puerperium

There are two separate but related phenomena that can occur following the birth of a child:

◆ the 'blues'
◆ puerperal psychosis.

The 'blues' defines a transient episode of low mood, crying, feelings of confusion and anxiety, intermingled with times of feeling happy. These symptoms tend to occur about the fourth or fifth day post-partum. Although the precise reason for this feature is uncertain, it may be caused by a rapid drop in hormone levels.

Puerperal psychosis, which has its peak in the month after birth, can still occur up to 2–3 months after. The aetiology of the psychosis is unclear but the risk factors associated with the disorder are:

◆ a family history or a previous episode of affective disorder
◆ not having a partner at the time of the birth
◆ perinatal death
◆ Caesarean section.

For women who have had a previous episode of puerperal psychosis there is often great anxiety about going through another pregnancy, dreading that it is going to recur. Regular support and involvement of the partner and family, along with counselling, may be helpful.

Parenting

Parenting is a complex task. At one level it constitutes a special form of relationship (see Chapter 10), at another it involves the provision of a rearing environment that includes reciprocal intimate play and conversation, as well as experiences that are needed for children's development. Amongst other things, this requires a sensitivity and responsiveness to children's cues; it also entails monitoring, supervision and discipline.

Many factors are likely to influence parenting but five stand out as particularly important.

1. Mothers and fathers bring to parenting qualities derived from their own upbringing and experiences of being parented.

2. Parent–child relationships will be influenced by the marital relationship. A person's relationship in one domain affects their relationships in other domains (Hinde & Stevenson-Hinde 1988).

3. The characteristics and temperament (as well as gender) of the child will shape the parent–child relationship. Parenting is a two-way process and the individuality of the child influences interactions and reponses.

4. Experiences will be important. Difficulties in conceiving or life-threatening illnesses may both lead to unusually overprotective parenting styles.

5. Becoming a parent is a very different experience for each person; for some it is eagerly awaited, for others it is a burden or stress.

In addition, parents tend to respond differently to their first-born child compared with later children. The relationship is usually more intensive (note the number of photographs taken!) but may also be more tentative and tense because it is the first. Usually parents become more relaxed with subsequent children so that the first child may later complain 'You never let *me* do that!'

Infertility

Infertility is an important life event that affects many couples. The prevalence rate is 15% for couples who have been trying to conceive for 2 years. Not all couples want children but procreation does have significance for both individuals and society (Clulow & Mattinson 1988).

The diagnosis of infertility can be a shock and give rise to confusion about the future and about hopes and expectations. It can affect the sense of identity of the individual and of the couple. It can seem to bar the way to a 'rite of passage';

Case study 11.3

Mr and Mrs Jones had been attending the fertility clinic for 14 months when they asked to see the counsellor. Mr Jones sat impassively leaning back in his chair, his body turned to look out of the window, whilst Mrs Jones sat on the edge of her chair, eyes wide open and breathing quite fast. Mrs Jones was eager to say why they had come explaining that 'this business' was getting them down. They kept having rows and he often went out with his mates to the pub while she stayed in unable to face her friends. She looked over to him and suddenly burst into tears and cried, 'I don't seem to be close to him anymore.' Mr Jones found it difficult to respond but eventually he agreed that this was coming between them. He said, 'She needs a baby more than me. It seems her only goal in life. We don't have fun anymore. Why can't we let nature take its course? I just want us to get on with our life. I don't want to go ahead with any more treatment; it's not getting us anywhere, we've been going for over a year now. There's lots of things we could do – just the two of us.' They finally turned to face each other and Mrs Jones said, 'I just need to keep trying – can't you understand that?'

The enormous gulf that had opened up and the conflict on how to resolve it was very apparent.

becoming parents and then grandparents, becoming truly adult, sharing a meaningful life with friends and other family members. The impact of these painful and powerful feelings can give rise to a sense of failure and a decrease in self-esteem. Tensions and conflict may arise in the relationship (see Case study 11.3).

Infertility is certainly psychologically very challenging, although for most couples it does not pose a psychiatric risk. The prior relationship of the couple is a key factor in coping (Pengelly et al 1995). Some couples are able to find a way of sharing the experience in that some women are able to carry and express the overwhelming emotion for both of them whilst the man copes with finding out about treatments and dealing with practicalities of appointments (Pengelly et al 1995). Sometimes couples do not achieve this balance and the distress may be overwhelming (see Box 11.3).

For many couples the greatest stress lies in their loss of control of a crucial aspect of their lives. It is an important part of human functioning to feel able to shape one's life and to direct life's trajectory – situations and events taking that away are experienced as threatening.

Infertility, like other stressful events, tends to accentuate pre-existing characteristics and relationship qualities, and accordingly it may have either positive or negative effects according to the success or failure of the coping. Many couples have to reappraise their life's hopes and expectations, providing the potential for growth. Some couples feel the experience has brought them close together and meet the challenge by exploring other ways of being creative. For others, feelings of failure, of being abnormal and of low self-esteem give rise to high levels of distress. These reactions are more likely in people who have previously experienced emotional difficulties, whose marriages are unsatisfactory and who lack emotional support.

Box 11.3 Risk factors for distress include:

◆ a strong expectation that fertility is synonymous with high levels of happiness, fulfilment and maturity.
◆ a continuing search for causal explanations of the infertility
◆ avoidance of the issues associated with infertility
◆ a loss of control in other areas of life, such as work or leisure.

Reflection point 11.1

Infertility is a good example of an experience that can serve either to close down or open up opportunities. How would you react to a couple concerned about infertility?

MID-LIFE TRANSITIONS AND EXPERIENCES

The term 'mid-life crisis' has recently entered our vocabulary, and appears to convey the notion that it is necessary to go through a phase of distressing and disturbing self-questioning. The concept is misleading, however, for two rather different reasons. First, it is normal to experience doubts and uncertainties about all transitions; the phenomenon is far from restricted to mid-life. Second, the questioning need not necessarily involve turmoil.

Transitions are considered here in relation to:

1. the 'empty nest'
2. retirement
3. grandparenthood.

The empty nest

The stereotype of the woman who suffers from 'empty nest syndrome' is misleading. Rubin's (1979) study showed that a great majority of women in their mid-40s viewed the departure or impending departure of their children with a sense of relief, albeit mixed with some ambivalence. Even so, it does not mean that it is of no importance. For some mothers, the departure may be a relief if the relationship was tense and unhappy, with the children's leaving having benefits for everyone. For other mothers, a feeling of loss may dominate when the child has been used for their own emotional needs. Usually, too, the departure may serve as a marker of a young person's independence and the need to adjust the relationship to a more adult footing. The child's departure may provide the mother with an increased independence to take on new responsibilities or make a career move, which may or may not be welcome. This transition is likely to have implications for the marriage relationship and this will very much depend on what has gone before. If the marriage has been dependent on the children, then their leaving may expose a rather empty relationship.

Retirement

Retirement is often viewed as a stressful event but research does not back up this stereotype (Warr 1987). The experience will depend on the person's personality and coping skills, past experiences of change and the social context in which it happens.

If retirement involves a move to a retirement home/community this change may feel distressing or difficult. Leaving old friends behind and having to make new friends or live in a strange place may feel like a loss of everything safe and familiar.

Box 11.4 Elements determining whether retirement is a positive or negative experience

Positive

◆ Retirement at the normal expected age is not necessarily stressful.

◆ When a job has been boring, stressful or very demanding

Negative

◆ A possible drop in income, bringing financial worry and a more restrictive lifestyle.

◆ Potential loss of status and work satisfaction. (There may be less stress if the person can still maintain some work interests or develop new ones.)

◆ Ill health coinciding with retirement, especially when expectations were of enjoying the rewards of a lifetime of work.

◆ Adjusting to longer periods of time being spent together with the partner. If the relationship has not been a particularly harmonious one then the time factor may be very difficult to negotiate. If both partners retire together the complexities may well increase further.

Life expectancy has risen markedly over the past few decades and many men and women have at least 30 years in the post-retirement phase of their lives. It is important that we do not classify all people over 60 years of age as old. Laslett (1996) argued that it does not seem appropriate to refer to this as 'later life' and for many people there is the 'third age' when people have energy to invest in many interests and activities. The onset of frailty is better thought of as the 'fourth age'.

Grandparenthood

In Western societies the average age for becoming a grandparent is about 50 for women and 52 for men and in some cases can be much earlier than 50. For example, a 28-year-old woman said, 'I could break my daughter's neck for having a baby. I've just got a new boyfriend. Now he will think I'm too old. It was bad enough being a mother so young – now a grandmother too!' To a large extent the role has changed in that grandparents are younger and frequently have their own work so that they are no longer available for full-time child care. However, it appears that most people welcome and enjoy the role (Smith 1991). Grandparents often feel a sense of emotional fulfilment and an evocation of feelings about their own parenting. Nevertheless, in about a third of cases there seem to be difficulties either relating to getting old, or over conflicts with their own children regarding child-rearing practices.

OLDER AGE

Moving into older age

There are cultures in which old age is regarded as the ideal, and is equated with wisdom and dignity so that older people are treated with respect. However, in our society there is a great deal of emphasis on youth, so that older people either feel or are seen by others as having reduced power, with consequent negative effects on self-esteem. Views on our changing biology have led to an expectation of declining health and competence in old age. Of course, there is an element of reality in these expectations. Extreme old age tends to be accompanied by failing memory, reduced vision and hearing, and restricted energy and mobility. But the stereotype is seriously misleading for four different reasons:

1. In most cases, the decline does not take place (at least in marked form) until a person is in their 80s and 90s rather than in their 60s and 70s.

2. There is huge individual variation in the effects of age.

3. Decline is much influenced by the extent to which individuals remain active physically and mentally.

4. Old age may bring new experiences with opportunities for growth and achievement. Personal development is as much a feature of later life as it is of other years (Baltes et al 1999, Wells 1999).

Everyone can think of people who demonstrate that old age can be a time of creativity and success. Grandparents travel the world, hiking mountains, gaining university degrees and continuing to do important work. Many older people find life more satisfying than at any other period of their lives and remain well adjusted, have a sense of control over their lives and maintain high self-esteem. On the other hand, many old people dread becoming frail and having to be admitted to a nursing home, which they fear will render them powerless to make decisions about their lives. Because illness is more common in old age, many old people fear that they will be unable to afford medical expenses in a nursing home, or to look after their ill partner. Loss of independence, loneliness, loss of status and reduction in physical and mental capacities are major sources of stress. It is obvious that people's skills in their use of coping strategies to deal with the changes of old age will be shaped by their previous coping experiences, their individual personality and their success or failure in dealing with earlier life transitions.

Vaillant's (1977) long-term follow-up study of Harvard university students from 18 to 65 showed traits such as perseverance, self-control and being able to see the bright side of life as important features for good outcomes in later life. Clausen (1991) also found that the ability to make competent choices in adolescence was carried over into later life enabling people to marshal, draw on and maintain social supports and achieve their objectives. Genetic factors also affect the ageing process and the individual variations that it shows.

Loss in later life

In later life the death of a spouse is a powerful stressor, giving rise to an increase in depression, and also mortality, during the 6 months following bereavement (especially in men). Men tend to keep themselves busy as a means of diversion from their grief, whereas women are more likely to want to talk (Lund 1989). Bereavement is most stressful when the surviving partner lacks other close social ties. Thus, older people are most at risk when they have lost many of their friends through death, moving house, or their children having moved away.

One of the most difficult experiences of grief is that following secret love, e.g. in a gay relationship that has not been socially recognised, or in an extra-marital relationship when the couple is unable to spend their final days together.

The ability to make new relationships for emotional support is very important. On the whole, men are less good at this than women, being less likely to have close, intimate, confiding relationships. It may be that because of this, men's initial reaction to bereavement tends to be somewhat more marked. A lack of spouse may force a complete change when the surviving partner cannot cope alone, which may mean a further change in moving to live with a son or daughter or going into an old people's home. The maintenance of social ties is very important for mental health; the existence of those ties, or the ability to make new ones, is crucial. This is likely to be a function of personal characteristics and of social styles developed in earlier life. For some people there is an enormous relief when the death of a partner brings an end to a long and painful period of dying. There may also be a relief when the relationship before death has been very difficult. However, when there have been ambivalent feelings in the relationship, feelings of guilt may appear. At this time the patient who needs help with the grieving process may also need help with the future – learning a new set of skills to cope with new responsibilities such as managing finances or household chores. For many widowers these are crucial to becoming competent, independent and regaining self-esteem.

CONCLUSION

It is curious how long it has taken for people to become aware of the developmental importance of transitions and experiences in adult life. The challenges and changes of childhood are crucial but so too are those involved in work careers, love relationships, cohabitation and marriage, parenting, grandparenting, bereavement and retirement. Each stage of life involves a mixture of continuities and discontinuities that is characteristic of developmental processes, and each provides the opportunity for enhancement or loss of successful functioning.

BIBLIOGRAPHY

Meerabeau L, Denton J (eds) 1995 Infertility: nursing and caring. Scutari, London

REFERENCES

Baltes P B, Staudinger U M, Lindenberger U 1999 Lifespan psychology: theory and application to intellectual functioning. Annual Review of Psychology 50: 471–507

Clausen J S 1991 Adolescent competence and the shaping of the life course. American Journal of Sociology 96: 805–842

Clulow C, Mattinson J 1988 Marriage: inside out. Penguin, London

Elder G H Jr 1998 The life course and human development. In: Lerner R M (ed) Handbook of child psychology, Vol. 1. Theoretical models of human development. Wiley, New York

Erikson E H 1950 Childhood and society. Norton, New York

Erikson E H 1959 Identity and the life cycle. Psychological Isues Monograph 1. International University Press, New York

Fagin L 1998 Occupational loss. In: Parkes C M, Markus A (eds) Coping with loss, BMJ Publications, London pp 70–80

Golombok S, Fivush R 1994 Gender development. Cambridge University Press, Cambridge

Hetherington E M, Lerner R M, Perlmutter M (eds) 1988 Child development in life span perspective. Erlbaum, Hillsdale, NJ

Hinde R, Stevenson-Hinde J 1988 Relationships within families: mutual influences. Clarendon Press, Oxford

Laslett P 1996 A fresh map of life, 2nd edn. Macmillan, London

Lund D A (ed) 1989 Older bereaved spouses: research with practical applications. Hemisphere, New York

Main T 1986 Mutual projection in marriage. Comprehensive Psychiatry 5: 432–449

Noller P, Callan V J 1991 The adolescent in the family. Routledge, London

Parkes C M, Markus A (eds) 1998 Coping with loss. BMJ Publications, London

Pengelly P, Inglis M, Cudmore L 1995 Infertility: couples' experiences in the use of counselling in treatment centres. Journal of Psychodynamic Counselling, October

Quinton D, Rutter M 1988 Parenting breakdown: the making and breaking of intergenerational links. Avebury, Aldershot

Rubin L B 1979 Women of a certain age: the mid-life search for self. Harper Row, New York

Rutter M, Rutter M 1993 Developing minds: challenge and continuity across the life span. Penguin, London

Smith P K (ed) 1991 The psychology of grandparenthood: an international perspective. Routledge, London

Taylor V J 1992 Pregnancy: a shared experience? Men's experiences and feelings about their partner's pregnancy. Journal of Advances in Health and Nursing Care 2: 59

Vaillant G 1977 Adaptation to life: how the best and brightest came of age. Little Brown, Boston

Warr P 1987 Work, unemployment and mental health. Clarendon, Oxford

Wells D 1999 Transitions: healthy ageing – nursing older people. In: Heath H, Schofield I (eds) Churchill Livingstone, Edinburgh

Wortman C, Biernat M, Land E 1991 Coping with role overload. In: Frankenhaeuser M, Lundberg U, Chesney M (eds) Women, work and health: stress and opportunities. Plenum, New York

12

The impact of illness on sexuality

Marjorie Rutter

KEY ISSUES

- ◆ Sexuality and bodily functioning
- ◆ Body image and sexuality
- ◆ Psychosexual aspects of specific illnesses including cancer, sexually transmitted infections and coronary heart disease
- ◆ Recognizing the sexuality of disabled people

INTRODUCTION

Illness and disability in all their forms may have either transient or lasting consequences for the emotional and sexual lives of people. This may come about through effects on self-concept as well as through the direct consequences of the illness, or of its treatment. Illness may be involved with loss – physical loss of a part of the body as well as loss of independence and privacy. Patients may feel inadequate if they have to rely on others for help with everyday living such as personal hygiene, dressing, or hair arrangement. Some drugs impair sexual potency and others may reduce sexual desire (see Chapter 5). The illness itself may have adverse effects either through influences on energy or mobility or through local effects on the genital organs. How individuals cope with these effects and the feelings they induce will be influenced by how they have met challenge and change in the past. The meanings they attach to the experiences will impact, as well as the responses of other people such as their partner, close family and friends. The impact of the illness is also likely to be affected by how the person is dealt with by professionals, not just in relation to the disorder itself, but in terms of their respect for the individual and their understanding of what the illness means for that person. Nevertheless, out of the distress and pain of illness can come pleasure and rewards through successful coping.

Because the focus of this book is on clinical practice in the field of sexuality, we do not discuss the many ways in which social and psychological factors influence people's vulnerability to physical illness. These are vividly illustrated in the Whitehall longitudinal studies, which show how rates of illness vary greatly by work circumstances, and especially by their implications for people's control over their lives (Marmot & Wilkinson 1999).

As outlined in Chapter 8, there is a two-way interplay between body and mind, but in this chapter the focus is on the consequences of illness rather than its causes. In this chapter particular aspects of sexuality related to illness and disability are discussed and specific body systems that are affected by illness are considered.

SEXUALITY AND BODILY FUNCTIONING

Body image and sexuality

Sexuality is often equated with physical attractiveness and the media do much to persuade us that we should 'keep young and beautiful if we want to be loved'. The ideal body is equated with youth and vigour as exemplified by the popularity of beauty and health clinics, saunas and salons and by the purchase of beauty preparations by the million. Operations, illness or injury may all impair people's body image because of the real or imagined loss they entail. At one time it was thought that disabled people who expressed sexual needs were in some way peculiar; the best thing a doctor could do was tell them to get these ideas out of their heads. Acceptance of this attitude was only a short step from believing that the disabled did not want sex and therefore had no sex problems (Greengross 1979). In response to this attitude a committee on Sexual and Personal Relationships of the Disabled (SPOD) was set up and, partly through the work of this committee, a change in attitude began to take place. It was recognised that disabled people have the same sexual needs as anybody else.

Body image reflects the way a person sees herself and how she is perceived by others, together with the values attached to these perceptions. Burnard & Morrison (1990) suggested that body image affects self-esteem. If people are content with their functioning and appearance they are more likely to feel generally good about themselves. For example, a young woman who had just had the diagnosis of blocked fallopian tubes said, 'I can't rely on my body now – my future seems to have changed overnight'. Her damaged body blocked off some of her key hopes and expectations.

Many people who are ill are likely to have worries about their own and their partner's sexual feelings. Assumptions should not be made that anxieties do not exist when the patient does not raise any concerns about sex. Lamont et al (1978) noted that partner education, acceptance and interest are important factors in the recovery of the sexual, as well as the physical, person. The partner may want to show love but be afraid of intimacy, fearing that they may cause problems or damage (Box 12.1).

Adolescents who develop chronic or life-threatening illnesses may be particularly vulnerable to fears about effects on their relationships. Some worry that they may be rejected sexually because they have a damaged body that others will find repellent. This may lead to either social withdrawal because they think others will not value them or, sometimes, promiscuity in an effort to prove they are still attractive. Physical dependence on parents may also be particularly difficult at an age when increasing psychological independence is expected. Worthington (1989) found that spinal injury and brain injury were particularly difficult for adolescents since it meant they constantly needed assistance at a time when they were trying to become independent. He also noted that when peers were unable to cope with the behavioural disturbances or changes in appearance, the isolation of the teenager increased. Adolescents with chronic illness remain dependent on their parents for longer and experience anxieties and uncertainties about their futures.

Van Ooijen & Charnock (1995) argued that, regardless of level of sexual activity or direction of sexual orientation, sexuality cannot be divorced from people's image of themselves in health and illness. At times of illness, sexual communication is often of special value for reassurance and restoration of feelings of personal worth as well as release of tension. It is important to get

---

Box 12.1 Effects of illness on sexuality

◆ Vulnerability implicit in the illness itself – how it is perceived, including the threat to the future and the fear of death and dying

◆ Helplessness, including loss of control of the body; invasion of the body by others and dependency on others for survival

◆ Altered body image, which may include distaste, feeling dirty, smelly, abnormal or unwholesome

◆ Anxieties about treatment and pain

◆ Guilt and self-blame for the possibility of having caused or contributed to the illness

◆ Anger and resentment – 'Why has this happened to me?'

away from thinking about sexuality only in terms of penetrative vaginal sex. Giving and receiving pleasure in different ways can be sharing, intimate and enriching and give positive reaffirming feelings. Being 'touchable' in any form is often vitally important (see case study below).

It is important to understand the feelings of dependency and powerlessness in illness so that whenever possible, the patient can be empowered to share in decisions about their own treatment and management. Solzhenitsyn (1988) said:

> *No sooner does a patient come to you than you begin to do all his thinking for him. After that, the thinking is done by your standing orders, your 5-minute conferences, your programmes, your plans and the honour of your medical department; and once again I become as a grain of sand, just as I was in the camp. Once again, nothing depends on me.*
> *(p xx)*

Although it is important to encourage patients to participate in decisions about their care there are times when pain and distress become overwhelming and this is not possible. It is then crucial that the practitioner is sensitive to vulnerable feelings so that these can be shared either by talking or by

Case study 12.1

Stewart, a young man of 24, was diagnosed with a brain tumour soon after he married Jean, and although the tumour was removed the prognosis was not good. Subsequently he became impotent, lost all his drive to work, felt inadequate and became totally dependent on Jean. Jean was overwhelmed by his dependency and did not know how to help him regain some of his independence. When she came to the clinic to discuss stopping her contraception she expressed anger about having to be 'his mother'. She desperately wanted him to be stronger in order for them both to be able to face his death. Stewart agreed to come and talk, and together they were able to negotiate ways in which he could take some control in their lives. He agreed to take charge of some tasks of home maintenance, doing business chores on his PC and taking care of meal plans which involved writing shopping lists for the helper. This meant that when Jean returned from work the surprise meal had already been bought and cooked by their helper. They enjoyed planning Stewart's new role and gradually he regained some of his strength and contemplated returning to work part time. For 3 months they rejoiced in his new found strength and gained enormous pleasure and intimacy from caressing. Although this was for a short period before his relapse, Jean described it as 'our summertime' and it had an enormous strengthening effect for them both.

physically being 'held'. Savage (1995) gives us a brief glimpse into an intimate relationship between nurse and dying patient: '... it was more just sitting on his bed. And he'd give you a look and just shake his head – it was a lot like that. Or he'd say, "Oh Jane," and reach out and hold your hand. He became quite sad when he wasn't crying. Then he'd swing into being quite happy.' In this instance, there has been fusion of bodily and psychological domains.

Recognising the sexuality of people with a disability

Able-bodied people tend to make assumptions about how disabled people feel, not recognising that they have sensuous erotic and sexual feelings. This may partly stem from assumptions that are held about the disabled person's body. Morris (1991) identified a number of stereotypical assumptions, i.e. that disabled people:

◆ feel ugly, inadequate and embarrassed
◆ crave to be normal
◆ desire to emulate able-bodied people in appearance
◆ have been affected psychologically because of their physical impairment.

Able-bodied people tend to hold views about disability that reflect only their own perspective and awareness. This readily leads to a chain of negative values ascribed to the disabled, involving putative psychological, emotional and intellectual characteristics. It is important to recognise just how much socialisation processes have led to discrimination against disability. In a study

Case study 12.2

Mr and Mrs Smith, a couple who both had cerebral palsy, requested help with contraception. Together, they decided that Mrs Smith would take oral contraception and would begin with her next period. We talked about positions that might be comfortable and they were excited at the prospect of feeling protected and safe. At the second visit all seemed to be well with pill-taking but when I enquired about sex they both hesitated and looked at each other. The difficulty they were experiencing was not with intercourse but with the other residents in the home. They had constant knocking on their door after supper, and when they did not answer, they felt that one or two had been standing outside the door listening to their love-making. The couple were aware that there was much interest in their sexuality and many questions were asked by other residents in an overt way that they found very intrusive: 'What do you do?' and 'How do you do it?'

using photographs where health workers were asked for their first impressions of people, results showed a positive correlation between physical attractiveness and attributions of personal characteristics such as being more cooperative, approachable and motivated (Nordholm 1980). Despite these negative stereotypes, many disabled people have a very positive perception of their bodies and it is this perception that matters. Others, however, have a negative perception and may feel unlovable and sexually unwanted. Some patients feel that sex will damage them and that they could be punished for indulging in sex. In some residential homes for people with disabilities there may be a particular focus on couples who are sexually active when the majority are not, as in the Case study 12.2.

Reflection point 12.1

Allowing patients to talk about their experiences gives both the patient and the professional new insights and ways of understanding and helping. What opportunities do you give your patients to talk?

SEXUAL ASPECTS OF SPECIFIC ILLNESSES AND DISABILITIES

Breast cancer

Maguire & Morris (1978) reported that one in four women undergoing mastectomy suffer anxiety/depression and one in three have sexual difficulties in the year following mastectomy. Such problems may become chronic unless recognised and treated. The meanings attributed to body parts are important factors in sexuality and the breast is a symbol of womanhood, motherhood and being sexually attractive. Sexuality may be seriously threatened by the loss or disfigurement of the breast. The distress may be increased by the diagnosis of cancer and the realisation of the life-threatening nature of the disease. Fallowfield et al (1990) reported that, for most women, the dread of cancer and possible loss of life is even more devastating than the fear for the breast.

It may be that some women feel guilty because they feel responsible for having caused their illness through an unhealthy lifestyle. Apart from breast surgery there may be unpleasant side-effects from radiotherapy, such as increased pigmentation and erythema. Effects from chemotherapy, such as hair loss, can be very distressing and some women develop amenorrhoea and loss of libido. A woman's partner, children and close family members will most

Box 12.2 Feelings associated with body image and cancer

- ◆ the body being eaten away
- ◆ something going out of control in the body
- ◆ something invading the good cells
- ◆ something unclean
- ◆ pain.

likely be affected by the illness and it is helpful if they can talk about their fears and anxieties. Partners often find it difficult to cope with their own fears of possible death or disfigurement, and while the woman may have an awareness of these feelings, both may find it difficult to share them. For both patient and partner a scar may seem very frightening and distasteful and as a result intimacy may be impossible. Some women attempt to avoid facing the reality of their loss by refusing to look at their chest, covering mirrors, getting undressed in the dark and taking less time with bathing. It is these women who are more likely to suffer depression and have anxieties about their sexuality.

One woman told the nurse that her sex life had been ruined because her husband said the whole thing turned him off. If breasts were an important source of stimulation before surgery, then it is important to help them both find alternative ways of enhancing pleasure in love-making. For some couples the trauma can bring them close together but for others there may short- or long-term problems. Studies have highlighted the importance that partners play in the psychosexual rehabilitation of women with breast cancer. When women present with sexual difficulties it is important to find out about the partner's response. Maguire (1985) found that those men who were able to provide affirmation of love and affection, and who prevented their wives from concealing their scars and/or encouraged sexual contact, greatly assisted the recovery of their partners.

Following mastectomy, all women are now offered a breast prosthesis of their choice and are encouraged to wear it within 2–3 days of operation. However, this may not necessarily be effective in alleviating distress.

Hysterectomy and cancer of the female reproductive organs

The uterus, usually has special significance for a woman's concept of herself as female. The loss of menstruation, and of perceived femininity, may negatively affect a woman's self-image so that she sees herself as sexually less desirable. To many women the thought of having a hysterectomy fills them with fear and dread and stories abound about 'never being the same again' or 'they take everything away and that's it'. There is also misinformation about what the operation entails – some women have a mistaken view that when the womb is removed the vagina is sewn up. It is clear that women need to have detailed information pre-operatively, know exactly what will be done to their body and have an opportunity to discuss fears. Tunnadine (1978) advocated that all women should explore *before* operation whether the removal may represent a loss of her emotional and sexual self. Some women come to hysterectomy eagerly, particularly if they have suffered from heavy, painful and frequent periods which have made them feel exhausted and never free to enjoy sex. For many of these women there will be a new lease of life and an enhancement of their sexuality. Others may hope their sexual lives will improve but not have their hopes realised and subsequently may find themselves feeling angry. It is important for practitioners to encourage sharing of fears and fantasies before surgery (Tunnadine 1978).

Shingleton & Orr (1987) suggested some questions that can open up a dialogue with patients:

◆ What does your womb mean to you?
◆ How will hysterectomy change your life?
◆ What is the most important function of your womb?
◆ What are your thoughts about losing your womb?

In other words what is the meaning of this operation for each individual woman?

When the uterus is removed for malignancy, fears of death and dying are likely to be present and need to be acknowledged. Younger women undergoing hysterectomy, particularly if they have not achieved or have not finished their family, may be especially vulnerable to the loss, and so experience feelings of emptiness associated with infertility.

As with other life changes, what has gone before is particularly important to adjustment. If sex has been satisfying previously, it is more likely that sex will continue after surgery. Supportive, understanding relationships with her partner, friends and health care workers are of great value. Womens' expectations of the operation may be self-fulfilling and those who believe that the operation will decrease their sexual arousal may secure their release from sexual relationships.

Tenderness may persist for about 12 weeks post-operatively, but couples should be encouraged to resume sex as soon as it feels comfortable. Different positions may be helpful in order to avoid abdominal or vaginal discomfort. Following the operation women may feel different sensations with intercourse, particularly if the uterus had been enlarged, hard, bulky or low-lying. Some women are aware of decreased sexual response because scar tissue may have formed in the vagina at the site of surgery or sensory nerve pathways may have been interrupted making tissues less sensitive (Wabrek & Gunn 1984). The character of orgasm may change because of the lack of uterine contractions. Not all women are in a sexual relationship at the time of surgery and single women may worry about their future sexuality without a womb. Lesbian women also need to be assured that love-making can continue to be pleasurable.

Cancer of the genital organs may be felt as shameful, particularly if the genital area has been thought of as secret, hidden, dirty and unspeakable. The psychosexual aspects of surgery of the ovary, cervix, endometrium and vulva are associated with loss of self-esteem, feelings of unattractiveness, loss of femininity, and sexual and other marital problems (Maguire & Morris 1978). Pre-operative counselling is important and the partner should be included in this process in order to explore feelings and expectations. It is also helpful for couples to be able to hear each other's fears and fantasies so that these can be acknowledged and shared. Talking about aspects of sex will reinforce the view that sexuality is not over, and ways of pleasuring that may not include sexual intercourse can be discussed. For example, there can be mutual masturbation, caressing of other erotic areas such as breasts and buttocks, and oral sex if vaginal sex is not possible. With any surgery to the genital area, appearance will probably be changed and help with self-examination is important.

The quality of the marital or cohabiting relationship has a most significant influence on recovery (Lamont et al 1978). With the diagnosis a woman is likely to be confronted with fears of death, and her partner is likely to feel threatened by this too. Lamont et al (1978) and Derogatos & Kourlesis (1981) reported that the most important factor in sexual rehabilitation is for the partner to be educated and involved.

Women may have similar fears to their partners and may convince themselves that it is impossible for their partner to desire them. Cairns (1983) found that about half of men suffered secondary impotence after their partners had gynaecological cancer.

Box 12.3 Partners' feeling about genital cancer

◆ Anxiety that the cancer could be transmitted by sexual contact
◆ Feelings of disgust and shock
◆ Fear of damaging or hurting his partner
◆ Anxieties about having a sexual life in the future.

Abnormal cervical smears and infection of the vagina

Cervical cancer accounts for 15% of all cancers diagnosed in women and often women blame themselves for this, linking it with early sexual intercourse and promiscuity. These factors have been highlighted in the media and some women believe that they are being punished for their sexual behaviour, leading to shame and guilt. Such feelings are aggravated when the women think that others are making such attributions. Studies have shown that these feelings may deter people from having a smear test (McKie 1993). Anxieties associated with an abnormal test result may include:

◆ fear of cancer and its consequences
◆ fear of pain in future treatment
◆ fear of having passed it on
◆ how did I get it? – which may be related to past relationships
◆ fears of damage to vagina and womb
◆ fear of diminished fertility and future childbearing
◆ feeling soiled and dirty.

All these feelings are likely to give rise to disruption of sexual feelings and when further tests or examinations are needed, such as colposcopy, the woman may feel her vagina is being invaded. Distress and anxiety can lead to a variety of responses such as anger, withdrawal, disbelief, confusion and guilt, all of which may cause difficulties in a relationship.

We should not necessarily group together all infections of the vagina as being sexually transmitted and it is important to be clear, when giving test results to patients, the nature of any infection. Many women, at some time, will have minor infections unconnected to sexual transmission but may, nevertheless, experience sexual anxieties about their vagina.

Doctors and nurses need to be alerted to women who repeatedly present with vaginal discharges but in whom tests are always negative. Unexpressed sexual anxieties may underlie these presentations. For many women the feelings surrounding a vaginal infection, sexually transmitted or not, may additionally involve concerns over the source of the infection, raising questions about fidelity, commitment and honesty of their partner. These feelings may continue and be difficult in future relationships. Unresolved anger and hostility may disturb future relationships, with feelings of mistrust giving rise to sexual difficulties. Many clients are anxious about starting new relationships when they have had genital herpes (see case study below).

Coronary heart disease and cardiac surgery

Myorcardial infarction (MI) is often thought of as a male illness, but more postmenopausal women die each year from MI than from breast cancer. Sudden

Case study 12.3

Amy attended the family planning clinic for a routine cervical smear. She told me that she hadn't used any contraception for about 2 years. When I asked further she burst into tears and said how worried she was about starting a new relationship. There had been lots of opportunities but she felt anxious and uncertain. As we talked further, Amy was able to verbalise her ambivalence about her sexuality. She very much wanted to have a relationship again and hoped it would be the 'right one' in which she could settle down and have a family. But she said, 'I'm very scared – I've really got to tell a partner that I've had genital herpes in the past and this could come back again in the future. I'm scared what someone will think of me. I've never been able to tell even my close friends that this happened and I still feel tainted and angry. He (her previous boyfriend) just clammed up when I got the result. We never talked about it. It broke us up in the end, I couldn't trust him.'

Reflection point 12.2

Amy's story highlights some of the feelings involved that get in the way of having a sexual life after a genital disease. Most women will recover a sense of equilibrium and recover their self-esteem, but some will remain vulnerable and need psychosexual help. How would you have responded to Amy?

death during sexual intercourse is often a great anxiety for men and women with a diagnosis of heart disease or hypertension, but such death is very rare. However, many people who survive MI suffer psychological damage that affects the quality of their lives by affecting their self-confidence and their sexuality. Some patients are still anxious and depressed and have sexual problems 1 year following the heart attack. They feel fragile and vulnerable and this dampens sexual arousal and contributes to a fear of resumption of sexual intercourse, which will have an impact on the partner and may lead to frustration.

Maguire & Parkes (1998) pointed out that the significance of the heart as a symbol and source of life may be the reason 'interference with the heart is likely to undermine our sense of the world as a safe place and of our body as a stronghold'. They suggest that cardiac surgery brings a realisation of the seriousness of their illness and is a cause of fear. The amount of distress pre-operatively correlates positively with post-operative distress. Many patients remain fearful of exerting themselves even when they have recovered good cardiac functioning, as the following case study highlights.

> **Case study 12.4**
>
> Jenny, a bright, young-looking 31-year-old, came to the family planning clinic after a gap of 12 months. She had been using the oral contraceptive pill but her last prescription had run out 6 months ago. She told me, in a rather irritated voice, that she had stopped the pill because her husband, aged 48 had had a coronary heart by-pass operation about 9 months ago. When I asked how he was, she said with very tight lips, 'The doctors have passed him "A1" and he's back at work.' However, her manner did not reflect the good news and I sensed that there was some problem. I asked, 'When are you hoping to start back on the pill?' She replied, 'Goodness only knows – I keep hoping something is going to happen. I tell him how fit he looks and I often get sexy but he never makes any moves. That's it – nothing is ever said.' We talked about her anger and frustration and she acknowledged that he was probably frightened although the doctors had told him he was fine. I wondered if they might share their feelings and understand how it was for each other. About 3 months later Jenny returned with a smile, asking for some more pills.

Practitioners need to be aware of the fact that male potency is often affected adversely by illnesses affecting the circulation and by their treatment. This applies, for example, to some of the drugs used in the treatment of heart disease and hypertension and it also applies to some of the consequences of diabetes. Medical care does not always include (as it should) a discussion of these features of illness and nurses may need to help couples understand what is happening medically (getting specialised medical input when required).

Skin problems

Skin is a very outwardly visible feature of a person and tiny blemishes and spots can cause a dent in our self-image. Many people invest a great deal of money and time trying to improve their appearance with creams and lotions in order to portray a picture of wholeness, freshness and attractiveness. People who cannot conform to this picture because they have skin disorders are more likely to feel dissatisfied with their appearance, unattractive, ugly and, possibly, repellent. There may be fears that others will think the problem is contagious, thereby avoiding close contact. This is a two-way process and a vicious circle of isolation, insecurity and feelings of unworthiness readily develops. Teenage acne is often a very emotionally painful disorder and may inhibit contact with the opposite sex because of embarrassment, being unclean or being repulsive to kiss. When the disorder is more permanent, it may make it difficult for people to start relationships. They may engage in heavy makeup and other techniques to disguise their defects at great cost to themselves both financially and emotionally.

Mental disorders

Mental disorders are exceedingly common; about one in three people will suffer from one over the course of their lifetime. Although sexual problems arising directly out of severe psychiatric conditions are likely to be dealt with by psychologists or psychiatrists, those associated with depression and anxiety impinge on nursing practice in the field of sexuality. Three features stand out.

1. People's mental states are likely to influence their interactions with others. When individuals are feeling low they tend to be irritable and bad tempered. It is a common occurence for the role of depression in deteriorating marital relationships to go unrecognised.

2. Libido is as much psychological as physiological. A diminution in sexual desire is frequent in depression (and a marked increase is common in mania, which is characterised by elevated mood).

3. Many drugs used in the treatment of mental disorders have occasional side-effects on sexuality. The class of antidepressants represented by 'Prozac', for example, may impair sexual potency.

Also, some drugs are associated with a tendency to weight gain, with the possibility of consequent effects on body image in relation to sexuality.

CONCLUSION

It might be thought that the impact of illness on sexuality is a rather specialised topic, requiring knowledge on all sorts of specifics regarding particular diseases. However, for the most part, that is not so. The experience of illness, both physical and mental, is something that affects most people at several points during their lifetime. As with other life experiences, how people cope with the challenges of illness will be influenced by their individual psychological style, by past experiences and by the ongoing interplay between body and mind. These themes all have strong influences on the impact of illness on sexuality.

BIBLIOGRAPHY

Bright R 1996 Grief and powerlessness: helping people regain control of their lives. Jessica Kingsley, London

REFERENCES

Burnard J, Morrison L 1990 Body image and physical appearance. Surgical Nurse 3: 4–8

Cairns K V 1983 Sexual rehabilitation of gynaecological cancer patients. SIECCAN Newsletter, Toronto, 18(1)

Derogatos L R, Kourlesis S M 1981 An approach to evaluation of sexual problems in the cancer patient. Cancer Journal for Physicians 31(1): 46–50

Fallowfield L J, Hall A, Maguire G P, Baum M 1990 Psychological outcomes of different treatment policies in women with early breast cancer outside a clinical trial. British Medical Journal 301: 448–551

Greengross W 1979 Acceptance of sexual feelings in the disabled. In: Lincoln R (ed) Themes in psychosexual medicine. Stuart Philips

Lamont H A, De Petrillo A D, Sargeant E J 1978 Psycho-sexual rehabilitation and exenterative surgery. Gynaecologic Oncology 6: 236–242

Maguire P 1985 The psychological and social consequences of breast cancer. Nursing Mirror 140: 540–547

Maguire P, Morris T 1978 Psychiatric problems in the first year after mastectomy. British Medical Journal 279: 963–965

Maguire P, Parkes C M 1998 Surgery and loss of body parts. In: Parkes C M, Markus A (eds) Coping with loss. BMJ Publications, London

Marmot M, Wilkinson R G (eds) 1999 Social determinants of health. Oxford University Press, Oxford

McKie L 1993 Women' views of the smear test: implications for nursing practice. Journal of Advanced Nuring 18: 972–978

Morris J 1991 Pride against prejudice. The Women's Press, London

Nordholm I A 1980 Beautiful patients are good patients. Social Science and Medicine 14A: 81–83

Savage J 1995 Nursing intimacy. Scutari, London

Shingleton H M, Orr J W 1987 Cancer of the cervix: diagnosis and treatment. Churchill Livingstone, Edinburgh

Solzhenitsyn A 1988 Cancer Ward. Bodley Head, London

Tunnadine P 1978 An age for concern. In: Lincoln R (ed) Themes of psychosexual medicine. Stuart Philips,

van Ooijen E, Charnock A 1995 What is sexuality? Nursing Times 91(17): 2–27

Wabrek A J, Gunn J L 1984 Sexual and psychological implications of gynaecological malignancies. Journal of Gynaecologic and Neonatal Nursing 13(6): 371–375

Worthington J 1989 The impact of adolescent development on recovery from traumatic brain injury. Rehabilitation Nursing 14(3): 118–122

Section 3

Coaching for psychosexual awareness

13

Participating in Balint seminars

Jane Selby

KEY ISSUES

◆ WHO definition of sexual health
◆ Gaps caused by uncertainty
◆ The Balint approach
◆ Workshops and seminars for tutors

INTRODUCTION

This section is written particularly for tutors and clinical managers who are keen to help their students or staff become aware of psychosexual issues and develop psychosexual skills. In these chapters some guidelines and suggestions are offered for those who are considering how to incorporate sexual care into their health promotion, health care and education programmes.

WORLD HEALTH ORGANIZATION DEFINITION OF SEXUAL HEALTH

It is now well recognised that sexuality and sexual health are integral to health. The WHO (1986) identifies three key components:

1. The capacity to enjoy and express sexuality without guilt and shame in fulfilling relationships.
2. The capacity to control fertility.
3. Freedom from disorders that compromise health and sexual reproductive freedom.

This definition clearly combines the emotional and physical components of sexuality, the essence of this book.

GAPS CAUSED BY UNCERTAINTY

Although sexual matters are recognised as being important, practitioners are often reticent about getting involved in this work (Waterhouse & Metcalfe 1991, Gamlin 1999). This situation has been reflected in education where programmes for health workers have generally had little to say about sexual issues. Scott (1995), however, thinks that 'a start is being made to remedy the situation'.

After even a brief training period educators may find their embarrassment can change to confidence; their feelings of not having sufficient knowledge change to an awareness that their knowledge is sufficient. They then become enthusiastic and keen to offer support for practitioners engaged in sexual care.

THE BALINT APPROACH

Many practitioners feel a lack of skills and want to increase these, in order to work with sexual issues of patients (Grigg 1997, Gamlin 1999). The method offered by the Balint approach could answer the requirements of educators who are undecided in their approach and recognise the need for some training. It offers ways to help practitioners become alert and aware of the psychosexual needs of their patients. The insights gained in a Balint seminar can encourage different ways of relating to patients.

In a seminar early examples of stories by practitioners usually offer a medical model of taking a patient's sexual history with questions and answers and little notice may be taken of the patient's way of replying or the behaviour. After studying encounters in a group, practitioners learn how they can try a different approach and feel supported.

The Balint seminar offers opportunities for:

◆ reflective practice
◆ clinical supervision
◆ action research.

In the training discussed here, emphasis is placed on the practitioner's skills of listening to the story, responding appropriately, and recognising the feelings that are evoked when meeting patients. Through the interaction and understanding of the practitioner–patient relationship psychosexual care can be offered. This training underlines the importance of incorporating psychosexual care into day to day work with patients and is applicable to all levels of clinical practice. The approach can be particularly useful for those who are already qualified and gaining experience in the clinical field. The practitioners have reached a stage in their work when they find themselves listening to their patients and wanting to offer help but feel inadequate in their responses. Then there is often a search by the professional for further skills and an appetite for training that is challenging and exciting.

The Balint training seminar is a small group of no more than 12–15 practitioners, coached by a leader (Randall 1992). During the seminar, a practitioner recalls the interaction experienced with a patient, and in a small group relives some of the feelings from that encounter. This becomes an important aspect for study by the group. A large group would be too intimidating, and the trust necessary to tell the full truth for this kind of work could not develop (Main 1989).

Teaching staff are often expected to impart knowledge to large numbers of students (Palmer 1998) and those educators who value small group situations may have to put a strong case for changing their approach. Whilst it may be possible to teach the human emotional development (Section 2) in a larger group, learning about human skills requires a small group.

Expectations of training

Practitioners attending psychosexual training seminars may be called upon to give sexual advice and counselling for a variety of patients. It is important for practitioners to understand that, when training in a basic level seminar (see Chapter 14), they should not be expected to practice as psychosexual counsellors. The skills offered at this level are for use as an integral element of patient care. Those who wish to undertake individual patient consultations need to continue training and to be supervised by attending an advanced seminar (Chapter 18).

Results of training

Students attending Balint workshops and seminars often say that it is the first time they have been offered perceptions and skills with which they can identify. Paradoxically, our experience is that many practitioners are already using these skills but are unable to recognise them for themselves (Benner 1984).

Attending Balint seminars is usually a stimulating experience and practitioners find themselves making changes to their practice. Rarely do members of a seminar group leave without some gain in awareness of psychosexual issues, but this experience is often quite painful and lengthy. Both leaders and students will need to recognise this. One member of a seminar group wrote:

The work is demanding but often rewarding for all (nurses, patients and leaders). Professionals, long grounded in prescriptive methods of patient care (do this and you will feel better), learn a new approach to problem-solving where the struggle is mutual; patient and practitioner together attempt to achieve clarity and insight. This is how the problems may be resolved or alleviated. Where there is an atmosphere of confidence and trust, the professionals and patients are drawn closer together in their search for insight. The seminar, for me, provides a new dimension of awareness in patient care.

The focus of study

The experiential framework offered by the Balint seminars, as described in these chapters, always has the focus on the practitioner–patient relationship for psychosexual work and the teacher–learner relationship for the development of teaching skills. This leads to a concentration on care for the individual patients, and contact with the practitioner provides the material for study in the seminar. The focus can be adapted.

Generalisation is not encouraged in discussion, as the study of a specific practitioner–patient relationship is the key to understanding the presenting anxiety.

The presenting anxiety is usually clarified as a result of the practitioner reflecting on a patient encounter, e.g. the patient appeared to be angry as he left the room after their meeting and the practitioner was puzzled by these feelings. The encounter is then brought to the seminar as an example of some discomfort in their relationship which had not been understood.

Many authors on reflective practice talk about a feeling of discomfort being the stimulus for reflection (Boud et al 1995). Practitioners may think: 'Why did I say that' or "How did I get into that mess?' As the practitioner–patient relationship is explored, the group members' comments often illuminate this reflection suggesting, for example, how the anger that worried the practitioner may be understood.

It is often a new experience for members of the group to present their work verbally, where no answers are offered or expected during the discussion. It is a way of negotiating the maze of a puzzling encounter.

The maze

In our experience, working with sexuality raises uncertainties, anxieties and confusion for all concerned. Schon (1987) provides a valuable insight into this:

In the varied topography of professional practice, there is a high, hard ground overlooking a swamp. On the high ground, management problems lend themselves to solution through the application of research-based theory and technique.

In the swampy lowland, messy, confusing problems defy technical solution. The irony of this situation is that the problems of the high ground tend to be relatively unimportant to individuals or society at large, however great their technical interest may be, while in the swamp lie the problems of greatest human concern. The practitioner must choose. Shall he remain on the high ground where he can solve relatively unimportant problems according to prevailing standards of rigor, or shall he descend to the swamp of important problems and non-rigorous inquiry? (p. 3)

Schon's (1987) insights are very relevant for this work. Meeting with patients and conversing with them at an emotional level is often difficult and cannot be solved by rational thinking alone. The Balint approach, however, offers a way of studying these difficult and often confusing aspects of care. With this approach it becomes possible to understand a situation through a mixture of 'feeling with', and 'thinking about' the patients' difficulties. This 'feeling with' allows the practitioner to perceive what a situation means to a particular patient at a specific time. When this meaning is more clear to both patient and practitioner, then they may think together about how the situation might be managed. Thinking can be very valuable if associated with a study of feelings.

Patients looking for help

Patients seeking help with their sexual lives rarely require specialist care but they do feel the need of a listening professional. The practitioner is not required to be a specialist but to stay with the patient and listen to what he wants to say at that time.

This very brief encounter illustrates the feelings of panic that practitioners often get when a patient expresses a worry about their sexual life. In the discussion that followed this story, several points were studied:

Case study 13.1

A practice nurse described in her first seminar a man who had come for a blood pressure check. She said, 'He is grey haired and has a beard. He comes to see me on a regular basis for his BP checks and sometimes sees the doctor for his prescription. I was taking his blood pressure and he suddenly said, "I have come in today because I am sweating when I have sex." I was so surprised, I had only seen him for 30 seconds, I felt I couldn't do anything, so I suggested he saw the doctor. Later I asked the doctor if he had said anything about sweating when he had sex, and he replied he had never mentioned anything about sex.'

◆ The nurse felt inadequate, didn't wait to hear any more and immediately suggested he should see the doctor.

◆ Patients usually choose the person they trust and wish to confide in. If they are referred to someone else the moment is lost and the distress has been missed.

◆ The patient did not choose to confide in the doctor and the moment of distress had gone. The immediacy of the problem for the patient had passed and the opportunity for the nurse to work in the here and now had disappeared.

Case study 13.2

A few weeks later the same nurse presented the story of a pretty young girl of 16 years old. 'I did not know her before this visit but she told me she was "itching down below" and could someone have a look. I suggested that I would do that if she liked. She agreed and she showed me her pubic hair which were full of lice. I told her what they were and she was appalled. "Where could I have got them from?" I enquired about her lifestyle and about her recent sexual life! I didn't panic.'

The second encounter shows the nurse working in the here and now – offering to examine the 'itchy area' and then being aware of the girl's feelings of being shocked on hearing the diagnosis. In the discussion the nurse said, 'I couldn't just leave it like that,' and then went on to explore with the patient where she might have picked up the lice. The patient's distress was not ignored. The nurse had started to develop some new skills in her psychosexual work.

The presentation of clinical material can be the starting point for the development of psychosexual skills, the creation of theory from practice and action research. The leader is there to coach and encourage the group to develop skills and make their own discoveries with the Balint approach.

WORKSHOPS AND SEMINARS FOR TUTORS

The following is a personal account of setting up a workshop and seminars to study a way of integrating sexuality into nursing and midwifery courses. I feel this experience could be a useful programme for other tutors or clinical management groups to consider.

The group was formed at the Avon and Gloucestershire College of Health (now the University of the West of England Bristol, Faculty of Health and Social Care). The Principal of the Midwifery School, Chris Tucker, approved and supported the project.

The project arose because, after many years of working and training in the field of psychosexual care, I became disenchanted with being invited to come as an 'expert' to work with nurses and other practitioners, giving lectures and workshops on the sexual problems of patients. They were usually one-off occasions and despite my asking if the course tutor would be able to attend, this rarely occured. The invitations were to lecture for 40 minutes or an hour and I always seemed to come at the end of the course. When I talked to the students they indicated that, apart from this session, the input on emotional care and sexuality was minimal.

Later on I became more confident and felt able to request time for a half- or full-day workshop, which I was granted, but I continued to come at the end! Most of the students were on post-basic courses, hence they were experienced and ready to develop new skills. The evaluations for my sessions were positive and had frequent comments like, 'I wish we could have had this earlier in the training'; 'Can we have more sessions?'; 'This day has been so relevant to my practice'; 'It has made me question my practice.' When I said good-bye to the group, usually after an interactive and stimulating time, I was aware there would be little or no follow-up of the lecture or workshop. This happened for two reasons, I think: it was at the end of the course and the tutors themselves felt they were too inexperienced to cover sexual issues. In the workshop situation, I felt the nurses had become more aware of their own and their patients' anxieties about psychosexual issues, but I was then leaving them in the lurch. The learning outcomes were minimal and there could be no development of the skills for which they yearned.

Initially I suppose I was flattered to be asked, I was aware I had some skills to offer and the response from the students reflected this. I seemed to be on the right track. I felt, and continue to feel, passionately that the sexual lives of patients cannot be neglected. My experience led me to realise that if I didn't do it, the subject of sexuality would not be covered in the course.

The attention given to emotional care has increased in recent years (Nichols 1993), which is demonstrated in practice, journal articles and books. However, sexuality remains the poor relation. I became convinced that this subject had to be integrated by the tutors in charge of the courses. Nichols (1993) suggests that 'improvements in the provision of psychological care within hospitals are, to a large extent, dependent on the nursing profession (although in some circumstances it is the therapist professions that are best placed to give such care).'

It was for this reason that I approached the Principal of the Midwifery School and offered to lead a short programme of training for tutors (lecturers now) to study a way of integrating sexuality into the curriculum. I used the Balint approach.

I knew that the tutors were unlikely to require knowledge about sexuality but they had evidently not found a way of working with the students' clinical experiences so that psychosexual skills could develop. If the tutors were going to use a Balint approach when teaching psychosexual care then first they needed to have the experience of reflecting on their own practice, i.e. teaching, in a group of peers. I devised a short course of two workshops and two seminars, based on reflection. In the workshops the tutors could explore the possibilities and problems in teaching psychosexual care. Then, having tried some discussion sessions with students, the tutors could reflect on these experiences during follow-up seminars. Both the format and the experience could become the basis of their own teaching of psychosexual care. These workshops and seminars could be organised in the future by the leaders of Balint seminars in the Association of Psychosexual Nursing. It is preferable if these are followed up with a regular 'tutor group'.

Philosophy

Psychosexual nursing/midwifery is an experiential training, and is the study of the professional feelings involved in working with clients' sexuality. It is not about the pathology of clients. Every client is unique, as are their anxieties. Each client's sexual life, needs and anxieties can be addressed as part of everyday clinical practice.

Aim

◆ To study and discuss the skills necessary for tutors to integrate training for psychosexual care into nurse/midwifery education.

Learning outcomes

1. The skills required for leadership are recognised by tutors.
2. To understand the importance of not necessarily producing solutions and to recognise there are often no 'prescriptive' answers.
3. To begin to recognise and use the nurse/midwife–client feelings present in each encounter.
4. The material for study comes from the student encounters with their patients.
5. To be able to integrate psychosexual care into any course or module.

Training time

Two half-day workshops (3 hours each) held within a month of each other; each had a formal programme:

1. To identify the sexual needs and anxieties of their client groups.

2. To identify the tutor's skills and anxieties in introducing sexuality into their curriculum.

3. To examine a way of helping students to work with clients' sexual care in their clinical practice.

4. To identify the feelings evoked in the nurse/midwife relationship with clients.

The workshops were followed by two seminars of 2 hours each, 4–6 weeks apart. This allowed time for the tutors to experiment with their student groups.

The tutors were asked (with no compulsion) to present and recount to the group their experience of introducing the topic of sexual care into the clinical practice of their students. The group would study each tutor's experiential work, reflect on the outcomes and evaluate the changes that they felt could be made. The presentation could be a group teaching session or about monitoring the skills of an individual student.

A short reading list was sent out before the training started.

It was agreed by the college and myself to invite all tutors in the college to attend. From a maximum of 12 people, 11 applied and 10 turned up for the first workshop. Some of the original members did not attend all the sessions.

In the event, tutors from two disciplines turned up: four mental health tutors and six midwifery tutors. I learnt at the first workshop that these disciplines had never had any connection with each other previously. I had met most of the midwifery tutors during my one-off visits but had not met any of the mental health tutors. It was a very experienced group who had mostly done their basic training in the 1960s and 1970s and had been tutors for a long time. Most of the tutors had little clinical contact with clients at the time except for two of the mental health tutors who also practised as psychotherapists.

The first workshop

At our first meeting we concentrated on the here and now, using the feelings that were expressed by the different tutors. I explained that all the work we studied would focus on the professional work of the tutors or students with patients. Their personal psychosexual problems and anxieties were not for discussion and remained their private property. As discussed in Chapter 14, this can be a relief for many tutors and enables them to maintain their professional role. One tutor arrived late, and at the evaluation time I asked him what that had felt like for him; initially he said, 'That wasn't a problem'; some of the group then said, 'But it wasn't alright for us, it felt quite awkward and we didn't know you'. We laughed and he admitted, 'It was difficult and I felt lost at the beginning.' We were then able to examine his behaviour in the light of how patients and students also feel about late arrivals.

The tutors found it difficult to offer their feelings, as opposed to their thoughts, in the discussions. This required constant clarification and 'teasing out' by myself; however, even the most experienced psychosexual practitioners find themselves expressing thoughts instead of feelings. It is one of the principles of Balint work to relay this difference to the students.

At this session, working in small groups, the tutors identified the psychosexual anxieties and needs of clients in their respective patient groups. These were recorded and discussed.

One of the psychotherapists raised a case he was seeing; it was an intriguing case but I had to point out that it was not appropriate to the focus of the day, which was to examine ways of integrating psychosexual awareness and care into their courses.

Many of the sexual anxieties of patients that were discussed were recognised in both of the disciplines and have been discussed extensively in this book. The mental health tutors were meeting more sexual dysfunction, lack of libido, sexual abuse and problems with sexual orientation. The midwives identified the effects of labour and childbirth on their clients' sexuality. Both disciplines were enlightened by listening to the different problems, but they were also able to reflect on their own previous professional experiences, vividly remembering these stories. This was considered particularly useful by the group.

The second question in the session concerned asking the tutors to share individual experiences of allowing clients to talk and share their feelings about these sexual needs. In the discussion the recognition of the importance of listening and responding skills in psychosexual work became evident, with the realisation that this can be therapeutic in itself. Particular reference was made to the initial assessment of patients and the need to enquire about their sexual health. The tutors also recognised the importance of discussing this with students early in their training to help them to incorporate this care into their daily practice.

Throughout the workshop I stressed that the material for study and learning can come from their students' encounters and stories. I am not sure they believed me! Before leaving I asked them to think of any changes that it might be possible to implement as a result of this workshop, if not immediately, perhaps in the future.

Second workshop

We met 3 weeks later, again for a 3-hour workshop. This time we looked at the tutors' skills and their anxieties about teaching sexuality. These were identified individually in writing and then I asked each tutor in turn to give me one anxiety or skill at a time from their list, until their respective anxieties had all been recorded on a flip chart for further discussion (Box 13.1). I pointed out that this is a very useful exercise – individual members of the group have to do the thinking and recording in silence. The tutors found it surprisingly difficult not to comment until the end! These findings then belong to the individual groups and the discussion, reflections and changes that may be implemented are theirs alone, which can be used as a chart to measure and identify the group progress in psychosexual care throughout any course.

Box 13.1 Skills and anxieties identified

Skills

◆ Able to draw feelings from students
◆ Comfortable with contraceptive issues
◆ Able to pick up non-verbal feelings
◆ Could draw from existing knowledge
◆ Not embarrassed
◆ Keeping a boundary within the professional role
◆ Empathy
◆ Use a variety of teaching methods
◆ Tolerant and open-minded.

Anxieties

◆ Fear of imposing own moral values
◆ Fear of not meeting student needs
◆ Worried by open interaction
◆ Lack of knowledge
◆ Not being an expert
◆ Constraints of curriculum
◆ Constraints of students offering sexual care
◆ Personal problems of students being brought out
◆ Supporting students with alternative views
◆ Coping with anger
◆ Dealing with homophobia
◆ The students raising issues I cannot cope with
◆ Selection of material for discussion.

These anxieties were discussed in detail and related to their present and future practice. Selby (1990) identified students' anxieties, and the similarity with the tutors' anxieties is marked.

People then began to share ways of working. Some of the tutors had been surprised how pleased their students had been to talk about clinical incidents they had encountered and were very observant and perceptive of psychosexual issues. They felt they had not been encouraged previously to discuss these openly or to reflect upon the incident. Some of the midwives felt they could work in pairs and run a workshop for their courses in the future.

By the end of the workshop the tutors felt that teaching about psychosexual care needed to be integrated from the beginning of their courses. Only then will this awareness of patients' sexual care develop alongside other skills that are being acquired. Remembering my own experiences, my message had always been that integration needs to start at the beginning of the course; there was now general agreement amongst the tutors.

Seminars

In the two seminars that followed, all the tutors were able to bring examples of integrating some of these ideas into their teaching. The tutors found it difficult to present in the beginning; some felt the work they presented was rather ordinary and I had to encourage them to remember the detail of the experience. Others said later, they felt quite embarrassed to show their own teaching practice and wondered if it would be acceptable to the group.

Practitioners have the same difficulties in their first seminars. However, as the tutors gained some insight into the approach, they were soon able to describe the setting and their teaching event. They came to value descriptions of what exactly took place, who was there and what happened. It was realised that without this description there could be no study. Feelings aroused in the tutor, whether with a client or students, were perceived as the crucial element for gaining insight into the client's or student's experience. In this short time we were only able to make a brief evaluation of the work. People from the two disciplines were most interested in the variety of teaching experience offered to their respective student groups. The Balint seminar was able to give insight into the individual tutor's initiative and the group reaction was stimulated by the discussions – an unusual and interesting experience for these tutors.

Evaluation

The evaluation of this experience was mainly positive but it was felt changes would be required for the administration as well as in the individual tutor's work. Rather to the tutors' surprise the project was enjoyable; for me, it was a stimulating experience and indicated the potential for change was there.

In a very small way I feel I have achieved my aim. This was recently confirmed as two of the tutors, now Senior Lecturers in Midwifery, wrote to say:

As a result of attending Jane's training seminars, we have been facilitating our own workshops with registered nurses who undertake modular courses in Family Planning and Cervical Cytology. For us, the seminars were timely; the need to explore issues of sexuality within our teaching was becoming increasingly necessary to enable nurses to focus more effectively upon the affective domain of client encounters. Without this experience of attending these seminars, it is doubtful that we would have found the confidence to faclitate sessions in a way that enables group participation and discussion.

The framework for discussion came from these seminars and provided us with a very useful approach in our workshops, and enabled us to facilitate them with confidence. Jane made us realise that we do not have to be 'experts' in sex and sexuality. This had been a major barrier to our belief that we were the appropriate leaders for such a workshop. The course members have enough experience between them to create a useful discussion. What we have are the skills to facilitate the discussion, maintain the focus and the ability to cope with what sometimes feels like chaos in the classroom.

We can honestly say, however, that there has never been a workshop in which we felt that we did not achieve our aims. Our skills have developed as we have progressed as facilitators.

Box 13.2 Main issues of evaluation

◆ The importance of focussing on the 'affective domain' in client care

◆ Having the confidence to use discussion seminars in psychosexual work

◆ The belief that one had to be an expert to talk about sexuality but now realising that is not the case

◆ Course members have the material for the study of psychosexual awareness and care

◆ Skills were developed to facilitate the discussion and maintain the focus.

REFERENCES

Benner P 1984 From novice to expert. Addison Wesley, Los Angeles
Boud D, Keogh R, Walker D 1995 Reflection turning experience into learning. Kogan Page, London
Gamlin R 1999 Sexuality: a challenge for nursing practice. Nursing Times 95(7): 48–50

Grigg E 1997 Guidelines of teaching about sexuality. Nurse Education Today 17: 62–66
Main T 1989 Training for the acquisition of knowledge or the development of skill? In: John J (ed) The ailment and other psychoanalytic essays. Free Association Books, London
Nichols K 1993 Psychological care in physical illness, 2nd edn. Chapman & Hall, London
Palmer H 1998 Exploring sexuality and sexual health in nursing. Professional Nurse 14(1): 15–17
Randall E 1992 Preparation for psychosexual nursing: results of survey of the ENB 985 at the Olive Haydon School of Midwifery – Lewisham Hospital. Goldsmiths' College, London
Schon D 1987 Educating the reflecting practitioner. Jossey Bass, London
Scott C 1995 Sexual health training in primary healthcare: a briefing of the Health Education Authority. Royal College of Nursing, London
Selby J 1990 Psychosexual nursing. Practice Nurse 3(2): 99–101, 112
Waterhouse J, Metcalfe M 1991 Attitudes toward nurses discussing sexual concerns with patients. Journal of Advanced Nursing 16: 1048–1054
World Health Organization 1986 Concepts for sexual health. WHO, Copenhagen

14

Setting up Balint seminars

Jane Selby

KEY ISSUES

◆ Setting up a seminar group
◆ Aims for the group
◆ Membership
◆ Setting
◆ Support in seminars
◆ Defence against work

INTRODUCTION

This chapter is in two parts. The first part shows how to start a Balint seminar group and the second part shows the progress of the group and the development of psychosexual skills for the members.

SETTING UP A SEMINAR GROUP

Tutors, clinical managers, or senior nurses may wish to set up a seminar group. When running the group it is preferable to attend a supervision group of leaders to monitor and develop the skills of leadership. The aims of the seminar should be to:

1. Present a story of a clinical encounter with the focus on psychosexual care
2. Develop a theory of practice
3. Explore with the group members the clinical events presented in the seminar.

Present a story of a clinical encounter

The basis of Balint training is the personal professional encounters told to the group and which are as important as the discussion and vital to the learning process. The encounters are the experiences of being with patients, the feelings involved and the emotional events that may have an effect on the situation (Section 2).

The opportunity to tell the story of one's own clinical work still seems to be rare for the majority of practitioners (Rafferty 1998). The story told by the practitioner in a seminar usually includes what happened between the patient and practitioner, the patient's concerns and how the practitioner felt about the encounter. The study in the group is then the practitioner–patient relationship. Unrehearsed stories are preferable to written records although a story may be chosen from a reflective diary.

Bowles (1995) writes about the appeal of stories in a nursing context. He cites the work of qualitative nurse researchers, such as Benner (1984), who are making use of 'lived experiences' to seek meaning within nursing practice. Stories heard in Balint seminars are indeed lived and living.

Develop a theory of practice

In the telling of and listening to stories during a Balint seminar, practitioners learn to tolerate the unknown, and to neither make assumptions nor offer reassurances. As a consequence new skills are developed in listening and responding to clues from patients' stories. The practitioner can then begin to work alongside the patient, to look at problems with mutual understanding. This also increases the practitioner's empathetic responses. The theory that evolves from these living and recent stories with reflective practice illustrates that practice can inform theory. As Schon (1987) suggests, 'in the unstable world of practice, where methods and theories developed in one context are unsuited to another, practitioners function as researchers, inventing the techniques and models to the situation in hand.'

Explore with the group members the presented clinical encounters

The supervision and support of the group and leader give courage to practitioners in their continuing psychosexual practice. The discussions are crucial to the progress of the group and the development of a practitioner's own aims.

Being close to the sexual distress of others is rightly seen to be difficult, sensitive and often painful work (Gamlin 1999). During the seminars the practitioners recognise and understand that human pain can be difficult to tolerate, but essential learning does emerge as the result of the work of the group and the leader. This is a gradual process; the required changes in practice come slowly, taking time and practice. Webb & Askham (1987) felt that nurses' rigid attitudes were likely to influence the quality and quantity of their relationships with their patients. Practitioners with little or no chance of supervision at their work, who as a result may have developed a certain rigidity of practice, can be especially disadvantaged.

The seminar leaders need to recognise and respond to the professional needs of each practitioner; this care for the practitioner can be offered as a model of patient care where the pain of the work is recognised and discussed with a possibility of an understanding (Chapter 6). As in all acquired skills, understanding needs regular and continuing practice. In relation to this, Main (1989) writes, 'Knowledge can be taught by a scholar to a pupil. Skill must be acquired – by daily practice with efforts to improve it.' It is the individual alone who decides what to do but they can be helped by a coach, the leader of a Balint seminar in this case, who can guide practitioners through the maze.

The importance of being in clinical practice while attending a seminar is illustrated below.

Case study 14.1

A tutor asked a leader if she could join a new series of seminars and explained her work was mainly in the classroom but she thought she could talk to some patients and have some clinical material for presentations. So, perhaps unwisely, the leader acquiesced, rationalising that this tutor might take back some of her learning to her own students. When the group began, all the members were in regular contact with patients and presented encounters for discussion and study – except this tutor.

As a result, the leader noticed the tutor become increasingly withdrawn and apparently isolated from the group. Crucially, the leader asked if the tutor was having any contact with patients, to which she replied that she now found she had not got time to talk to patients as she had hoped and she realised the importance to the members of maintaining clinical practice with this approach. The result was that, with mutual agreement, she left the group. The tutor admitted to feeling acute discomfort in the seminar and, indeed, the experience had been difficult for all. There was a sense of relief for the leader when the tutor left, and the group perceived that her departure was appropriate as she had been unable to present. The group also commented that they had felt constrained by her presence because there was no feeling of co-equality. It was only after the tutor had left that the leader noticed the group becoming cohesive and the work progressing.

As shown in the above case, initiation into Balint-style work needs to take place with a group who feel they are peers. The tutor profiled was unlikely to learn within the original group, but may have been more successful in a tutors' group (Chapter 13).

A lonely prophet's voice

Nearly 40 years ago, Abercrombie (1960) experimented with a course of discussion groups. She hypothesised that 'we may learn to make better judgements if we can become aware of some of the factors that influence their formation.' She found, 'The main difference between this and the traditional methods of teaching is the amount of attention that is paid to the *process* of observing or thinking, as distinct from the results. In traditional teaching the student makes an observation, and finds it to be correct or incorrect by comparison with the teacher's (or currently accepted) version. In the discussion technique of teaching, the student learns by comparing his observations with those of ten or so of his peers.'

In a Balint seminar the individual's way of working can be observed and a range of observations offered. As a result, their clinical practice becomes more flexible. Abercrombie's findings are supported by those who have trained in Balint seminars (Randall 1992).

The focus of study

Focus is on the psychosexual issues that the practitioners meet in day to day clinical work, and the care that can be developed. We have found that the word 'psychosexual' can disturb patients, educationalists and practitioners. It is therefore vital to define the meaning as used in this context. When discussing this work, Skrine (1997) refers to the 'intertwined nature of bodily and emotional pain'. The unravelling and exploration of the psychosexual pain and pleasure in sexuality is studied to allow the practitioner to increase the skills required to work with patients and their sexual concerns.

Main (1989) clarifies this meaning and writes, 'Sex is something more than body matter, more than bodily acrobatics; it is also a matter of high passionate feeling and the giving and getting of intense bodily and mental pleasure in the most intimate relationship of all. The sex act is therefore above all psychosomatic, and practitioners because their work involves touching and talking are in an ideal situation to offer psychosexual care.'

For practitioners in their professional role there are many opportunities of having contact with mind and body, which may not always be concerned with the sexual act but with other aspects, such as the patient not 'feeling their usual sexual self'. This feeling can be related to:

◆ self-image
◆ feeling dirty with incontinence
◆ having a stoma
◆ feeling unloveable after 'mutilating' surgery
◆ following a medical diagnosis of diabetes
◆ heart failure
◆ suffering from asthma.

All these feelings can be encountered by health care professionals during the daily care of patients in childbirth, cervical screening, urinary care, treatments in genitourinary medicine, washing, bathing, pre- and post-surgical care and medical care, including the care of the dying. During intimate care, the practitioner can listen and respond to overt and covert messages from the patients and the interaction between practitioner and patient can become a therapeutic event.

Membership of the group

The group consists of between 6 and 14 members and needs to be sustained for 1 or 2 years, with 18 seminars a year of 1.5–2-hours each. The duration can be flexible, but for permanent change to take place, members will need to attend between 30 and 36 seminars on a regular basis and remain in clinical work (Main 1989).

Shorter courses can be integrated into specialist practice and do not require the same strength of commitment since the aim is to make students aware of psychosexual concerns. After a short series of seminars, students often seek training in other seminars and continue to develop their skills.

The group members are co-equal, professional practitioners, each bringing their different expertise, specialties and skills to the seminar training. Practitioners usually attend because they feel inadequately trained in their awareness of psychosexual anxieties and care of patients' sexual lives, whether patients are ill or healthy (Box 14.1).

Box 14.1 Factors in group membership

1. There needs to be a feeling of commitment to learn new skills within an experiential learning framework.
2. All members of the group have to be in clinical practice, i.e. meeting patients on a day to day basis.
3. Where it is appropriate, the use of bodily examination is studied, which reinforces the body–mind approach.

Suitability for training

It is important that where the training is available the educators and clinical managers are familiar with the aims of a Balint seminar. It is not recommended that students are merely sent on the training solely because there is availability, a vacancy and/or money. It is important that the time is suitable for the practitioner to undertake this training. If the practitioner is experiencing a stressful time, such as bereavement or loss related to separation or termination of pregnancy, they may feel too vulnerable to undertake this way of working. Some practitioners will delay their training, whilst others may wish to seek some therapeutic help for themselves (Chapter 6).

The setting

All that is required is a quiet room where there is no disturbance, and chairs arranged in a circle. The initial atmosphere is set by the leader and should be felt to be a purposeful, working group. The leader's role is to coach and supervise only; it is not a didactic role.

The seminars should be held at a regular time and in the same room if possible. It is curious how important this is. The following story illustrates the difficulties when this does not take place.

Case study 14.2

The seminars were held in a school of nursing and the staff knew the time and day booked for each meeting. However, each time the leader arrived, the venue was different and invariably there were not enough chairs. Members arrived late because they had gone to the room previously used, so the leader had a dilemma as to when she should start. Inevitably – irritatingly – they always started late, but as they had to finish on time, each session was always curtailed. For the leader and the group, the situation was thoroughly unsatisfactory. The work seemed to lack purpose and the group developed poor time-keeping. The leader decided they must start on time and established with the authorities that the same room would be available in the future. Once the leader stopped waiting for latecomers, some group members soon realised that if they were late they had missed part of an encounter, making them feel excluded and unable to participate in the discussion.

When the leader established her authority appropriately, the group began to flourish. This story mirrors the encounters with patients, and the significance of a time discipline. The mutual control of the environment in which the encounter takes place can allow a fruitful practitioner–patient relationship to develop.

PROGRESS IN A SEMINAR

Introduction

Progress in a seminar is not only measured for the group as a whole but also for the individual members. People learn in a variety of ways and at different paces. Some are quick but impetuous, leaping into the discussion without much thought (perhaps that is how they work with their patients?). Others are thoughtful or guarded and tend to react more slowly. However, those who are able to be thoughtful usually make progress. Randall (1992) noted in his research findings that 'those who pursue an active interest in psychosexual work often possess a personal and professional maturity. Substantial professional and life experience seem to provide a good basis for seminar training.' In addition to a professional outlook, some of these experienced practitioners present most of the encounters on which the group is dependent for its study, and therefore its progress. A group's learning curve is not a steady rise but has peaks and troughs like a barometer; thus, the leader acts as coach to guide the practitioners through the confusions in this field.

Sharing

The word 'sharing' here means the telling of a story and the attentive listening of the group. Feelings expressed by the practitioners, whether in the initial presentation or the discussion, are respected. The leader establishes the atmosphere, allowing sharing of the practitioners' professional work.

During the first few weeks of a seminar the leader will observe which group members are anxious (Chapter 15). Benner (1984) suggested that practitioners move through stages of expertise, starting with being a 'novice', and this stage is re-experienced in each new field of practice undertaken. When joining a psychosexual seminar the practitioner is often exploring a new way of working and therefore feels the vulnerability of a novice. There is often, however, surprise and some relief from realising that others in the seminar have similar feelings (Endocott 1989). Until this is shared each may remain alone with the vulnerable novice feeling.

Sharing gives a common purpose and diminishes early anxiety, so that the process of beginning to work can take place, both individually and collectively. As the group develops, practitioners are enabled to reveal the secrets about their failures and successes in their professional lives. Group norms are gradually established (Wright 1989).

A member of a group recalls the feelings encountered when attending seminar training:

Initially mainly apprehension, inadequacy, curiosity and a slight foolishness. But for me this quickly turned to interest, clarified and stimulated new ideas as well as giving me fresh insights into psychosexual care for my patients ... But the main gain for me was the feeling of understanding and support given by all the group. In short, I felt safe and supported to develop new skills.

The cohesiveness that develops gives a sense of commitment to the group and can be experienced by each of its members. There is a commitment not only to the task and the leader but also to each other. The commitment is based on empathy, trust and understanding, as well as the positive support and security which comes from within the group. When this is recognised, it is an indication that the group is working well and beginning to achieve the aims of the training. They are no longer novices. Wright (1989) suggests, 'The sense of belonging to something that one values and which is valued by others produces a sense of worth.' Practitioners not only begin to grow new skills in psychosexual awareness and care but also grow more confident in their professional lives.

Presentation of encounters

Early presentations by practitioners are too often like a medical history report, limited to the patient and the problem, the family history and investigations. The practitioners are anxious that everything should be in order and correctly told. These early presentations are sometimes complicated, difficult and may indicate the anxiety of the practitioner, unconsciously asking 'how and where do I start?'

Case study 14.3

'Mrs D is a 42-year-old woman with multiple sclerosis, she is married for the second time and has two of her own teenage children. The doctor asked me to talk to her about a sexual problem to see if her problems were menopausal and whether HRT might help. On closer questioning, I learnt her husband worked late, had a meal, watched TV and sometimes a video as well and then went to bed late. Mrs D goes to bed early, often tired, and she feels their sexual relationship was suffering. I asked if they communicated, "Not really" she said.' Aside to the group, the nurse said 'but I have met him and he does seem to be caring and concerned about her condition.'
He continued with the story, 'I suggested early morning or daytime sex, she replied that no that was not possible the children might hear or see them. I felt I should be helping, as the doctor had asked me to talk to her, but I was getting nowhere. I gave her an advice booklet we have on the unit, dealing with multiple sclerosis and sexual problems, hoping she would raise the problem with her husband.'

Case study 14.3 was presented by a senior charge nurse on a Young Disabled Unit.

The following difficulties are shown in this encounter:

◆ The description of the woman was correct, but bland.

◆ She was referred by a doctor – perhaps he was hoping the problem would be cured by a prescriptive treatment but also felt unable to discuss the problem.

◆ Mutiple sclerosis is often a long, difficult disease to live with and there seemed to be no emotional exploration of her needs.

◆ The nurse was anxious to help and started to ask questions but was answered by negative replies. With this rebuff, he then offered a book.

In the seminar discussion that followed, all these thoughts were noted – but where were the feelings in this nurse–patient relationship? There was no description of the patient's appearance or where the encounter took place. The nurse admitted he had not really thought about any feelings but he reflected on the event and commented, 'I felt so overwhelmed by the task the doctor had set me, it all seemed to become too difficult, and at the time it seemed easier to offer a book.' He really felt he wanted to help this couple. The feelings that were expressed by the members of the group in the discussion were frustration, isolation and sadness. This was a revelation to this nurse, who then realised these were his feelings as well. The group wondered if he had made an assumption that the couple wanted to have sexual intercourse, whereas since the feelings were of sadness and loneliness perhaps Mrs D would have liked to talk about feeling alone and wanting to be comforted and touched rather than having sexual intercourse. The nurse thought he would try to share these feelings with Mrs D by saying, 'I felt some sadness and loneliness when we talked – I wonder if that is how it feels for you?' That could then lead to her revealing the feelings of loss which seem to have arisen with her illness.

Caring for people's sexual lives and the feelings that go with this care are always difficult, and to be able to start to talk and work with these is an enormous change for many practitioners. It requires courage. Previously the practitioner may have felt the need to suppress these thoughts and feelings. During the discussion of the previous encounter the leader had encouraged the nurse to tell the story as a clinical event, describing the patient's appearance, the setting of their meeting and a description of what had happened between them. That pattern quickly becomes the way of telling a story. In the second seminar a very different presentation was given (Case study 14.4).

The group then had a picture of this meeting and in the discussion they could study the behaviour of the patient and the practitioner, and explore the reasons for the patient's anxiety and tears.

A practitioner working in a well woman clinic described Helen: 'She was in her mid-40s, well dressed in a smart green suit and she told me she was working as a head teacher and it was very stressful. I felt she was anxious and tense but she seemed to be very much in control of the situation. I asked how I could help, and to my surprise suddenly the tears began to flow.' The sad story was heard.

Initially, the members will ask questions and expect answers because this has been the pattern of communication in the past (as seen in the first encounter). As this technique is repeated by others, the practitioners begin to understand that they do not seem to be helping their patients, and they do not seem to make progress, so the feeling is one of 'getting nowhere'.

The leader is responsible for making sure that the group continues to move forward and make the necessary changes towards becoming listening and observing practitioners, allowing skills to develop. The leader must also keep the group focussed on what happened in the encounter, what it felt like to be with the patient under discussion and on the practitioner's behaviour.

After further discussion the nurse involved in the first encounter began to see he had not got at the thoughts and feelings of Mrs D. When this understanding is reached in a seminar, it is possible to begin to accept and allow thoughtful silence, waiting for the patient to speak. With a change of approach, communication can become more productive. Patients may need help, e.g. the practitioner in the second story opened the conversation by asking, 'How can I help?' The practitioner may encourage patients to talk by enquiring, 'I wonder what you are thinking?' or 'How do you feel at the moment?' thereby giving space to the patients to express their own thoughts and feelings. Sharing of experience can then become the beginning of a working relationship between two adults with the ability to gain some insight into the problem.

An experienced health visitor illustrated this working relationship in her description of meeting Linda, a young girl with a new boyfriend (Case Study 14.5).

In the discussion that followed this encounter the health visitor described how she had felt very much in the 'hot seat' saying, 'Before I started seminar training I wouldn't have allowed Linda to express her worry, let alone discuss it. I feel I now have the confidence to try to listen to what she was saying. I tried to exclude *my* ideas and feelings, and tried to share *her* fears and worries. She had chosen to share her worry with me at that particular time and I tried to respond to her need.'

Case study 14.5

After a brief introduction the health visitor described her meeting with Linda. 'She suddenly said, "I really want to see someone about my sex life." I felt panic stricken. I told myself to relax and just listen to Linda. I asked her if she would like to talk to me about it. Linda launched into top gear and told me that she thought she had never had an orgasm and her boyfriend thought she should. She seemed eager to talk and I felt almost "taken over". We discussed what she knew about orgasm, it emerged that her boyfriend was very satisfied with their sex life but worried that she was missing out. On the other hand, she was enjoying love-making more and more. I remarked that they obviously had a loving, caring relationship together, and we thought about whether an orgasm mattered to her. Was it necessary to have one to achieve a measure of sexual happiness? She thought probably not and as she left seemed to be relaxed and excited.'

In Linda's story the acknowledgement of the patient's feelings in relation to her situation and telling the truth to the health visitor allowed the patient to feel she had been helped, and her anxieties allayed.

As the group progresses they begin to realise that a cure is not what they expect to hear from individual practitioners' encounters and they rarely hear of a perfect ending. There is a realisation that to join with the patient, and to find the truth about the patient's situation, may be all that is required and is therapeutic in itself. Many experienced practitioners as they progress in the training begin to realise that earlier forms of communication, such as making assumptions or giving reassurance, may not have been very effective – a humbling experience.

Learning may only be achievable intermittently and members early in training may feel they are not making progress at all. Gradually, as encounters are discussed, the practitioners realise that, providing a failure is understood, then to fail is okay. The work is not judged as being good or bad; each clinical event is studied for its own merits. As members relax they feel more able to report on their own feelings. Discussion becomes valued as an honest critique of presented work and, although it may sometimes be painful, it should never become a destructive process for any member of the group. This experience does not just touch the presenter but is felt by the whole group and the learning from the seminars will often be stored away for use in future patient encounters.

Case study 14.6 illustrates a woman's sexual distress and the discussion that followed in a seminar.

During the discussion, the group were initially enthusiastic and went off in all directions, generalising about sexual abuse. The leader had to bring them back to discuss this patient and this nurse's encounter. The presenter

> ### Case study 14.6
>
> Mrs B was well known to a school nurse, as her children had bed wetting problems and one child had a handicap of the hand. Mrs B was also the nurse's patient in a family planning clinic where she had recently confided that sex was pleasurable for her with self-masturbation but she had never had 'an accident'; on enquiry from the nurse as to what that meant she said an orgasm. The conversation that followed was not exploratory and the nurse remembered it being rather unsatisfactory.
>
> One day, Mrs B made a telephone call to the school and asked if this nurse could come and see her as soon as possible. The nurse immediately thought there must be some problem with the children, and made an appointment for the next day. She arrived to find there was no need to ring the bell as Mrs B was looking out of the window, obviously waiting for her. The nurse described her as rather wizened and wispy, old for her years; she was 32. Mrs B then told the nurse her father had died post-operatively 4 weeks ago and this had triggered some memories. The nurse said she felt quite annoyed at that stage. What was all this urgency about?
>
> Mrs B went on to tell her she that she had been thinking about her childhood. 'You know what I told you, I wonder if this has anything to do with that?' She remembered her parents going out one day each week and leaving her with a 'man friend' of theirs. She remembered wearing no clothes, sitting on his knee and enjoying that experience. She now wondered if that was abuse and asked the nurse, 'Do you think that is why I have never had an "accident"? Since my father's death I have felt much happier with my husband.'
>
> She had an appointment next week in the family planning clinic but said, 'I couldn't wait to tell you, and anyhow I wasn't sure that was the right place to talk to you again.' The nurse said she felt quite shocked by these comments and internally wondered if it was the father who was the abuser.

was surprised at her own reaction as she said, 'I am used to dealing with abuse in my work in the school but I have never met anyone who has told me this as an adult.' The group drew attention to Mrs B's control over the nurse, asking her to come to the house for her personal problems. As the group explored this nurse–patient relationship the question was asked, 'Was this control an indication of her relationship with her husband?' This apparently wizened, older-looking woman was perhaps internally angry with her father and his death had been a release from their 'hidden secret'. One member suggested that 'the practitioner's irritation with Mrs B seemed similar to the woman's own feelings and might well come from the patient's world.' The nurse felt 'that could be true' as the discussion explored this practitioner–patient relationship (Chapter 6). Another member said, 'She trusted you and wanted to confide in you again', while still another thought-fully said, 'but you never enquired about the story of the "man friend". Was this a fantasy or a fact?' The man friend was never discussed with the patient and 'this funny little woman's control' seemed to get in the way. The nurse remembered she had tried 'to discuss the bereavement' but the woman was quite calm and declined the offer. The leader also encouraged the presenter to remember her departure in more detail. She then remembered she had been offered a cup of tea but refused, 'I was so relieved to get away!'

This story and discussion illustrates some important points about progress in a seminar:

1. Work in the seminars is concerned with distress and changes in patients' sexual lives.

2. The reason for bringing an encounter is because this distress is not understood by the nurse or the patient.

3. Mrs B's distress had been a 'secret' but she chose to share it with this practitioner.

4. The nurse in this encounter was unable to share and give back that pain to Mrs B because of her control, but the learning for the group, as the result of the discussion, was that the pain always belongs to the patient and not to the nurse.

5. The discussion produced many different thoughts and opinions from the group members.

6. The encounter was painful to listen to, but this was shared by the leader and the group.

7. The nurse felt supported and there was the knowledge that the leader and group would continue to support her.

8. Individual practitioners' styles and defences become clear to other members and thus themselves.

9. One of the practitioner's defences here was to go into the questioning mode and little unravelling of this complex problem took place.

10. Members of the group observe the attitudes and behaviour of each other and can therefore make an honest critique.

Support in seminars

Support from the leader and the members in a Balint seminar allows practitioners to feel valued as professionals, giving them courage to work with patients' sexual lives. Many people flourish in this atmosphere, where there is a feeling of being nurtured. It is the offering of encouragement, as well as the hearing and acceptance of praise and admiration when things go well, that allows them to bloom. One seminar member commented:

I have a feeling of an intensity of concentration in the seminar and devoid from the rest of the world. With the focus on the case encounters at the time and afterwards I feel quite mentally drained but also stimulated. I felt I became more involved once I had made a presentation. It was testing but I felt the support of the group. Personally it has given me confidence to tackle situations that otherwise I would have backed away from.

Defences against work

'Defence' refers to the attitudes, social or temporal changes and behaviour that are common to us all, but are devised for the protection of the practitioner's personal and professional anxieties rather than for the primary care of the patient. It is not the purpose of the seminar training to explore the practitioners' personal defences although there is a recognition that they are part of the professional self (Chapter 2).

In a seminar the encounters reveal that sexuality is affected by many different scars, physical and emotional, both hidden and open. Gill (1989) writes, 'Because of their profession and training doctors can be said to have a "common core" of defences', and she goes on to say, 'some of these will be shared with other professionals, such as nurses, teachers and social workers.' It is not surprising that practitioners defend against patients' pain. In the Balint seminars, defence has been identified as an attempt to control the pain and discomfort for both the vulnerable practitioner and the patient.

Patients' defences

Defences can also be devised by patients for their personal protection. These defences are observed with increasing interest by practitioners as the training progresses, and can offer an important insight into the patient's troubles and distress. The practitioner often feels 'blocked' and helpless as an offer of help is rejected, e.g. as felt by the nurse when Mrs B did not wish to talk about her bereavement.

Sometimes patients may say, 'I can't stay today, I must fetch the children from school' or 'I'll make another appointment', but the appointment is never made. 'I don't know' seems to be a common reply heard by many practitioners, which may indicate that the thoughts and feelings of the event are too painful and difficult to recall. The practitioner may be able to encourage the patient to tell the story by saying, 'It seems to be difficult for you to remember what happened, perhaps it was very upsetting?'

Where an intimate examination is offered, e.g. a cervical smear, the practitioner may notice a warning sign of anxiety when a patient says, 'I haven't washed myself' or even 'my feet smell and you won't like that'.

These comments may be a challenge to the practitioner – i.e. 'don't you dare try' – or are an indication of the patient's embarrassment and used as a defence, fearing the physical and intrusive examination of a cervical smear. Before attending seminar training these remarks and excuses may not have been thought of as significant but with study the practitioner realises they cannot be ignored. Defences deserve respect; they may be life preserving for some. For patients it is their choice alone, whether or not they wish to reveal an anxiety. If the defence is understood then the question can be asked, 'Having revealed the problem, does this patient want to work with it?' Mrs B, despite revealing her problem, did not appear to want to go any further.

Practitioners' defences

Defences of both practitioner and patient can be difficult to spot in an encounter. Laughter and tears can be used, as well as denial and forgetfulness, by both patients and practitioners. Practitioners may also feel a lack of knowledge; they may not voice this lack but their behaviour can express it. Clifford's (1998) observations are that, 'Under the stress of not knowing how to respond to a particular difficulty, and without appropriate support it can be easier to regress to "knowing best", which requires less thought and effort.' It is often easier to return to the 'high ground' (Schon 1987) but as the practitioner becomes more experienced it becomes possible to cross 'the swamp' and listen to the beliefs and thoughts that come from the group and leader to understand these defences. The nurse caring for Mrs D felt he did not know enough and defended against this by offering a book and was therefore not able to offer space and listen to Mrs D (see Case study 14.3).

The use of physical examination can be of great value. It may help both patient and practitioner to understand an anxiety or a fantasy. Sometimes when a patient requests a physical examination a practitioner will say, 'I'll ask the doctor to have a look' or 'Yes, I'll come back and have a look.' The patient referred on to the doctor may never say what they wanted to discuss with the practitioner (Chapter 13) or the practitioner who says, 'I'll come back', sometimes forgets. Practitioners learn in the seminar that each of these responses may be a defensive move. The moment is lost, and may never be repeated. When a practitioner suggests a physical examination, it is important that she asks herself, 'Why am I doing it now?, Have I got a reason or is it that I cannot think of anything else to do?'

If examinations are conducted with sensitivity and thought, patients' anxieties and fantasies are often revealed.

Practitioners working in the caring professions are usually compassionate people but this can lead them to avoid patients' pain, fearful that if this is acknowledged the patient may break down. Trying to be kind and reassuring to avoid the pain may be the practitioner's defence against the knowing of this pain. Patients can be powerful with their defences and the practitioner may feel unable to confront this feeling. Practitioners' defences are often demonstrated by offering advice, reassurance, a book, referral, asking patients to bring their partner or by making another appointment. In the seminars the practitioners study their behaviour asking '*why*' and *how* did I do that?' Defences are often revealed as a control mechanism, masking uncontrollable feelings of confusion when the practioner feels helpless. Then she retreats from the work impotent and unable to think clearly. There is no insight into the practitioner–patient relationship. When the practitioner is aware of her own and the patient's defences she is more able to make choices about her own intervention.

Case study 14.7

The practitioner described Jenny, a pretty young woman coming to the surgery and complaining of feeling depressed since her termination of pregnancy 9 months previously. Before she was able to say anything Jenny collapsed into 'almost effortless crying; it seemed to last for a long time'. Eventually Jenny was able to tell the nurse that her mother did not know of the termination, or that the young man who lived in the house as a lodger was the father of 'her child'. The practitioner said, 'I felt distressed with the situation and at a loss as to how to help. Jenny started to cry again as she went in to see the doctor.'

In Case study 14.7 the practitioner had this feeling of helplessness, and was confused by the tears and the story; she was unable to think what to do next.

The discussion that followed explored the clues that Jenny left with the nurse:

◆ this was a painful story seemingly witheld until now
◆ the effortless tears – although distressing, were they a release?
◆ there were secrets in this family
◆ the loss of 'her child' seemed to be overwhelming.

The nurse had felt pain in this story but had been unable to understand it and was at a loss at how to proceed. The group uncovered the nurse's pain and recognised it came from Jenny's feeling of helplessness, loss and a strong request for a solution. The nurse was exhausted by this encounter. This encounter had a profound effect on the group for their future work. Tears and losses could never again be ignored and were recognised as valuable clues to a patient's anxieties.

The development of skills

The seminar is an emotive experience and at any time it is a turning point for the practitioner to start to experiment, explore and offer new skills to help patients. The quality of patient care is enhanced by this growing confidence and awareness of their patients' sexual lives. It is not a rigid learning experience and the time and space allowed in a Balint seminar is an essential part of its success. In the growth and progress for the practitioner, it can be painful having to lose well tried and old skills to make way for new skills. 'There is no growth without pain and conflict; there is no loss which cannot lead to gain' (Pincus 1974) epitomises the growth for the practitioner. The group members learn how loss, with all its pain, causes so much distress in patients' sexual lives, but with their new found skills there can be gains for their patients. It is important for the leader to allow the group to define these new skills, often verbally at the end of each seminar or when writing their seminar accounts. It is equally important for the leader to write up her own experiences of learning to run groups to monitor her leadership skills.

Box 14.2 Outcomes of learning in practitioners' seminar (from reviews of seminars, unpublished evaluations 1981–1999)

1. Ability to listen and recall

◆ Enhanced listening skills

◆ Listening sensitively to the verbal and non-verbal clues for the hidden need or distress behind the account

◆ Allowing the encounter to develop spontaneously rather than be guided by a detailed history

◆ Listening and thinking, using silence and observation rather than asking questions

◆ Accepting not always having to respond and have an answer

◆ Observing what interventions were used, the response from the patient and the effect

◆ Observing what interventions were thought about but *not* used

◆ Tolerating confusion and lack of understanding rather than feeling a lack of skills

2. Recognition of the practitioner–patient relationship

◆ Noting the meeting and the farewell of an encounter

◆ Recognition of the interaction in this relationship and the emotion evoked

◆ Examining the timing and mode of the presentation to the practitioner

Box 14.2 Outcomes of learning in practitioners' seminar (from reviews of seminars, unpublished evaluations 1981–1999) (contd)

◆ Noting the appearance, the manner, and behaviour of the patient

◆ Recognising that the emotions arising in the practitioner during the encounter could indicate the patient's difficulty

◆ Ability to accept and tolerate pain coming from the patient without giving reassurances

◆ Enabling the patient to see that solving the anxiety belongs to them and is not the sole responsibility of the practitioner

◆ Noting the changes that take place in the relationship during the encounter

◆ Recognising the private and personal life of the practitioner plays no part in this relationship

◆ Ability to recognise those patients whose difficulties are beyond and outside the practitioner's field of work

3. Recognition of the defences

◆ Being aware of the patient's defences and the reason for their use

◆ Identifying methods used to avoid discussing the anxiety

◆ Recognising the individual practitioner's defences

◆ The recognition of the practitioner's flight away from work by giving directive advice

4. Use of physical examination

◆ The ability to use the examination at an appropriate time and for an appropriate reason

◆ Being able to use examination therapeutically to throw some light on the patient's anxiety

◆ Being able to observe and recall how the examination was conducted

5. Participation by the practitioner in the seminar

◆ A willingness to participate in the discussions

◆ Presents relevant encounters and honest accounts of the work

◆ The ability to introduce relevant ideas and support the train of thought behind them

◆ Shows continuing interest, which can be silent and thoughtful

◆ To show an ability to enquire of each phenomenon, 'What does this tell me about the patient?'

◆ The practitioner is willing to accept and offer a critique of presented encounters.

REFERENCES

Abercrombie M 1960 The anatomy of judgement. An investigation into the process of perception and reasoning. Free Association Press, London

Benner P 1984 From novice to expert. Addison Wesley, Menlo Park, CA

Bowles 1995 Story telling: a search for a meaning within nursing practice. Nurse Education Today 15: 365–369

Clifford D 1998 Psychosexual nursing seminars. In: Barnes E, Griffiths P, Ord J, Wells D (eds) Face to face with distress. Butterworth Heinemann, London

Endocott J 1989 Coping with psychosexual problems. Nursing Standard 42(3): 29–31

Gamlin R 1999 Sexuality: a challenge for nursing practice. Nursing Times 95(7): 48–50

Gill M 1989 Defences in doctors. In: Skrine R (ed) Introduction to psychosexual medicine. Montana, London

Main T 1989 Training for the acquistion of knowledge or the development of skill? In: Johns J (ed) The ailment and other psychoanalytic essays. Free Association Press, London

Pincus L 1974 Death and the family. Faber, London

Rafferty M 1998 Clinical supervision. In: Barnes E, Griffiths P, Ord J, Wells D (eds) Face to face with distress. Butterworth Heinemann, London

Randall E 1992 Preparation for psychosexual nursing. The results of a survey of the ENB 985 at the Olive Hayden School of Midwifery. Goldsmiths' College, London

Schon D 1987 Educating the reflective practitioner. Jossey Bass, London

Skrine R 1997 Blocks and freedoms in sexual life. Radcliffe Medical Press, Oxford

Webb C, Askham J 1987 Nurses' knowledge and attitudes about sexuality in health care – a review of the literature. Nurse Education Today 7: 75–87

Wright H 1989 Group work: perspectives and practice. Scutari, London

15

Supervision of practice

Jane Selby

KEY ISSUES

- Group training
- Material for study
- Developments in groups
- Group behaviour
- Dissolving the group
- Leadership skills
- Training and support for the leader

INTRODUCTION

In this chapter the art and skill of leadership in a Balint seminar is considered. It is useful to have some idea of group theories before starting to lead a group. These theories show that a pattern of behaviour emerges. It is helpful to have participated in a Balint group but, for some, this may not have been possible, so this chapter will introduce tutors and clinical managers to the role that they could aim to take. The aim is to help students to give accounts of their own practice, and to support the group in studying these accounts for the development of insight and skill. It is a coaching role.

GROUP TRAINING

The theories to be discussed are particularly appropriate to experiential learning. Dr Michael Balint produced a fundamental change in the training of health care practitioners by emphasising the study of the practitioner–patient relationship, thereby involving practitioners in the emotional care of patients. Balint's system offers a pioneering way forward for those involved in training practitioners, i.e. practitioners bring recent examples of their practice to a group of peers for discussion. This work is difficult and requires skilled leadership. Teachers in health care are usually very experienced in group work, but they may not have studied the life of the group or their skill development when leading groups. It is important to obtain supervision, preferably in a group or alternatively on an individual basis (Chapter 13).

Whichever method is used, leadership skills can be developed more readily when the same disciplines of reflection and writing are used in the leader's supervision as are encouraged amongst the students attending Balint groups. The theory of groups will be discussed here but cannot replace the reader's own reflective work on their leadership.

The leader will need to reflect on each seminar. Writing up each seminar allows more than just time for recording who was present, absent or arrived late, but also for recalling the encounters that were presented. It is useful to keep individual evaluations of the students' progress, a reminder of the outcomes of learning that have taken place, the attitudes of practitioners and notes on their changes of practice. Experienced leaders find it advisable to complete this as soon as possible after each seminar. It is easy to forget the events and much can take place in a seminar of 2 hours. These notes are useful as an aide memoire before starting the next seminar, and are a private reflection and assessment of the work of the leader.

The good group experience

Group leaders hope to 'develop in a group the forces that lead to smoothly running co-operative activity'. Bion (1961), defining the 'good group experience' wrote, 'It is as hard to define as is the concept of good health in an individual', however, good groups do have common qualities (Box 15.1)

Group experience in a Balint approach

When using the Balint approach for the development of psychosexual work the following aims and boundaries should be added:

1. The material for study is experiential, using psychosexual encounters from the practitioners' everyday practice.
2. The study is of the practitioner–patient encounters and the relationship that is evoked.
3. The members work from ignorance of the unrehearsed encounter, as does the leader.

> **Box 15.1** Qualities of a 'good group'
>
> ◆ A common purpose
> ◆ Common recognition by members of the group of the 'boundaries of the group'
> ◆ The capacity to absorb new members and to lose members without fear of losing group individuality, i.e. 'group character' must be flexible.
> ◆ Freedom from internal sub-groups
> ◆ Each individual is valued for the contribution to the group and has free movement within it
> ◆ The members have the capacity to face discontent within the group and have the means to cope with this
> ◆ The minimum size of the group is three. With two members there are personal relationships; with three or more there is a change of quality to interpersonal relationships.

4. The leader is non-didactic.
5. Each group develops its own theory of practice by trial and error.
6. It is *not* a therapeutic group for the personal problems of individual group members.

The setting

The setting can be arranged in a professional ambience – on the ward, in a clinic, health centre, GP practice or an educational centre. It is essential to protect both the time and the space so that participants can attend the whole seminar without interruption. Without this protection the study of encounters is jeopardised. Seminars have been held in private homes but the temptation in the home is for the group to gravitate towards becoming a social gathering.

Time and length of training

Experience has shown that a 2-hour seminar period is best but, failing that, 1.5 hours has been used and allows just enough time for the presentations and discussion.

The group usually meets fortnightly, sometimes weekly. In the early days of learning it is important to keep up the momentum of study – weekly or 2-weekly seminars help the student to reflect on the seminar work and implement new skills in everyday encounters with patients. Monthly seminars can be held for more experienced practitioners.

Non-didactic teaching

The leader's role is to supervise and coach only, with the aim of allowing the group to acquire skills. Leaders try not to instruct, but require practitioners to think for themselves. Main (1989) writes, 'Didactic teaching, however good, has hardly any effect on the process of liberation for practitioners to start new ways of working.' Those educators who are experienced tutors and well trained in teaching from a knowledge and research base, may find some difficulty in changing to this approach.

One of the skills of leading a group is to instil a sense of co-equality and of working from ignorance, as in the satisfactory practitioner–patient relationship. Ignorance here does not mean ignorance of human life and its frailties but it does mean that each time a meeting takes place between a practitioner and patient it is unique; neither of them knows what will happen, and the work is then conducted in the here and now. Main (1989) writes of this practitioner–patient relationship: 'it is much more one of equality, co-ignorance and co-endeavour.'

Material for study

The material for study comes from encounters between the practitioners in the group and their patients. Significantly, experience has shown that encounters need to be recent – ideally, a meeting within 2 weeks of the seminar presentation. With time, recall fades and the ability to feel the atmosphere declines as memory of the detailed interaction dims. The story becomes less vibrant and therefore lifeless, less worthy of study within the context of experiential learning.

Leaders should not present encounters because then the material belongs to the leader and not to the members of the group. The leader's presentation would then detract from the practitioners' material, which is the 'initial subject matter' (Dewey 1974, p 364, cited by Schon 1987, p 16). It is also important for the practitioners and leaders to understand that the care of those patients who are suffering from mental health problems, often within complex disordered lives, is usually not suitable material for a mixed group of practitioners. These specialist practitioners will require their own group and may require a different focus of study where this approach can be used equally well (Griffiths & Leach 1998).

DEVELOPMENTS IN GROUPS

All groups have a life, a beginning, a middle and an end, which can be compared to meeting a patient, followed by the work, then the parting. These stages become significant for the group and leader as psychosexual encounters are studied.

The beginning

During early meetings of the group there is usually anxiety and even panic. Some students may wonder if this is the right course for them because they are unsure what will happen and who they can trust. Here there is an important role for the leader. The leader needs to show her awareness of the difficulty for the students but should not seek to take it away. An approach often used is for the leader to acknowledge the students' discomfort or anxiety and, when it is appropriate, point out this experience, since it is often similar for patients who want to explore their anxieties. For readers who are beginning to train with this approach it is useful to record how they work with the practitioners' anxieties.

As trust develops, an early group is characterised by dependence on the group leader. This is normal but the hope is that the group becomes more independent as it develops, and is then able to make its own discoveries from studying examples of practice. Early meetings can be a testing time for the leaders and when new to this work some have commented, 'I felt tempted to give them the answers.' With the support and supervision of a leaders' group a different way of working is encouraged and it is recognized that there are sufficient skills in a group without being told what to do. Telling group members what to do usually reinforces their dependency and therefore reinforces 'childlike' behaviour. The leader may find Eric Berne's formulation of transactional analysis helpful for their understanding (Chapter 3).

Erikson (1965) suggested that, in the life of a group, 'we are allowed many chances to rework issues which remain unsolved.' This recurring opportunity allows the group to trust each other and to work cohesively towards acquiring and developing new psychosexual skills.

The middle

The middle period is the work time. There may be uncertainties, unrest and even revolt as new ideas and thinking are discussed. Although the group is sufficiently cohesive and trusting to tell of their work, to listen and try to understand and offer insights, nevertheless there still may be a return to dependency. However, these difficulties have to belong to the group to allow them to gain confidence, develop skills and try them out, and to reflect again. Initially, groups may not always meet with success, and to continue this work usually requires stamina and an emotional will, as well as the beginning of respect for the task. Patients who come for a consultation make difficult and sometimes impossible demands on the practitioner, leaving a feeling of incompetence and impotence. The need to solve the problem then becomes the practitioner's burden. The leader needs to value students' skills, competence of care and compassion offered to patients as they progress in this difficult work. The leader will also need sustaining as she struggles to help practitioners develop a new dimension of emotional and sexual care. A leaders' group can offer this sustenance and allow patient, practitioner and leader to benefit from 'emotional labour' (Smith 1992).

The parting

The ending of a group is the parting of professional colleagues who have struggled together with the pain and pleasure of each other's work. They have usually become a cohesive group, offering support and supervision to one another, which has been described by previous members of psychosexual seminars as being a 'privilege' to have had the opportunity to share the experience. When patients leave the practitioner, however brief the consultation, it is hoped that the patient will also leave feeling they have been allowed to share their anxiety. They have shared sadness, pain or pleasure but the important aspect is the co-equality of working together to allow some insight into the presenting problems.

GROUP BEHAVIOUR

Bion (1961) described a group as having two aspects:

1. The Work Group, which indicates the aspects of the group prepared to work by confronting the painful and difficult issues that arise.

2. The Basic Assumption Group, an aspect of the group that is anxious and can display a variety of unconscious ways to *avoid* the work when it is painful and difficult.

Bion identified three common reactions of groups when they are obstructed, diverted or overcome by powerful emotional drives for avoiding work, describing them as 'dependent', 'pairing' and 'fight and flight'.

Dependent

Dependency may be particularly noticeable at the beginning of a group. The group is anxious and uncertain how to behave, as joining a new group is always a new experience. Initially, the leader may find the practitioners are resistant to 'the process of liberation' (Main 1989). An added difficulty is the study of psychosexual issues, which continue to be embarrassing and felt to be too intimate to recount in a group. The group, in this case, may wish, albeit unconsciously, to provoke the leader to become an expert and to offer answers, rather than studying the issues for themselves. In order to face the potent emotional issues some groups believe they need a 'deity' who will provide the solutions.

Consequently, the members do not always share their thoughts and skills to avoid the work task. If leaders collude with the group, then their role becomes one of taking charge. High value is flatteringly given by the group to the leader's comments, which are then considered more useful and appropriate than the contributions from the group members. As a consequence, the comments of the members may appear to have little value and are therefore ignored by the other members.

Groups can move away from this dependency: Bion (1961) suggests, 'groups get stuck there or will return there, usually because of their own insecurity and need for protection'. The leader may comment on this 'feeling stuck' feature and say something like, 'I am wondering if this work is frightening some of you?' The group then has a chance to voice their insecurity and continue their development of skills.

Pairing

Pairing is noted when two members of the group work together, sit together in the group and hold a discussion between themselves rather than with the others. This phenomenon can often be observed between two members and may be imitated by other members. The pair appear to ignore the rest of the group, rendering the other members impotent. Pairing may be a conscious or unconscious event, and may be observed as a way of competing with the group, perhaps implying 'we know more than you do'. As a consequence, the dependence of the group is centred on the pair to do the work, with the effect that others find it difficult to enter the discussion. Withdrawal takes place and the task of the group founders.

Fight and flight

The basic assumption here is that the group is meeting either to fight or to run away from the work task. Case study 15.1 illustrates running away from the work and the leader's intervention. The leader can also be a target, when the demands on the group may provide an opportunity for the group to be aggressive and in revolt. If members feel their comments or contributions are ignored they can involve the group in fractious behaviour and undermine the leader's authority. The fight could be between the leader and a member, or between two members.

The leader has to be aware of this behaviour, refuse to get involved, but study the battle, always leading the discussion of the group back to the presenting encounter in the here and now. The tendency otherwise is for the group to start talking in general terms or offering anecdotal contributions.

Supervision for the leader can help identify the group behaviour; even when the leader feels the group is progressing there may be a hiccough which

Case study 15.1

An experienced practice nurse described to the group an encounter with a young mother of three children, the youngest 2 months old. On enquiry from the nurse, she said everything was fine since the birth, but she had been told she should come for her post-natal visit by the health visitor. When the nurse enquired about birth control, she immediately replied she 'didn't need that now' and left without seeing the doctor. The nurse, glaring round the group, said, 'What do I do now?' The leader was aware of a flashing eye at her as well, as if to say, 'I do try, this is not working for me, I challenge you.' During the discussion the nurse said, 'I have always asked about birth control', implying that she did that well. (You will notice the nurse had returned to the generalisation and away from specific study of the young mother and their meeting.) At this point, the leader intervened and asked her to think about the woman's reply, thus bringing it back to the encounter. The leader knew she had heard the client's response as she recounted it to the group, but before the subsequent discussion there was little insight and no enquiry as to what the patient meant. The nurse felt the emotional task of enquiry was all too difficult and she did not want to get involved. The patient and the group had challenged her skills during the discussion and, on reflection, she realised she could have tried another approach which might have allowed the woman to share her problem.

needs understanding. This help may not be immediately available but a leaders' group can draw attention to this for future occasions. Dainow & Bailey (1989) comment, 'Many groups progress sequentially while others move backwards and forwards from one stage to another'.

Case study 15.2 illustrates one member of a group making a request to generalise, and the role of the leader in preventing this happening.

The leader asked for one encounter and the study became focussed on this one encounter which led onto other unique encounters. Each event was recognised as being contributory to learning. There was no flight from the task at the end of this seminar.

Tuckman (1965), after reviewing many articles dealing with groups, described a group as progressing through four stages:

◆ forming
◆ storming
◆ norming
◆ performing.

Case study 15.2

At the beginning of a seminar group of midwives, the leader asked who wished to present. There was plenty of work but one midwife said she would like to talk about examining perineums: 'I have lots of women who seem to have problems.' The leader responded, 'Can you tell us about *one* of your clients you have seen recently?' While the midwife thought of an appropriate encounter, the group studied other encounters and when it came to the time for the encounter on perineums, the midwife described visiting a specific client at home in the immediate post-natal period. She knew that this client was experiencing some pain but was very reluctant to be examined. The midwife persevered, explaining why she would like to examine her, and the client consented. While doing this examination she was able to share the patient's feeling of discomfort but the midwife left feeling uncomfortable.

The discussion that followed centred on the case and the discomfort of the midwife only. This specific focus led on to three other midwives describing encounters they had met in the last week, but without any generalisation.

One encounter was easy and comfortable for both client and midwife. The second occurred in the home with a father and mother. When the midwife found the father peering over her shoulder as she examined the perineum, she was surprised but enquired if he would like an explanation. The response was positive, there was no embarrassment and both the father and mother expressed relief at hearing that the lump they had found earlier was a small haemarrhoid. The third encounter followed a water birth. The midwife described the mother as resting comfortably on a mattress with her legs abducted and the perineum appeared to be totally open. During the seminar discussion the midwife said she felt quite shocked and described it to the group as 'looking like a motorway'. Initially her internal thoughts were. 'How does she have satisfactory sexual intercourse?' a very honest reporting.

Forming

Forming is described as the beginning of the group, when there is a need for dependency, orientation, trying to understand the method, the focus, the time boundaries as well as testing the leader's abilities to run the group. It is a time of uncertainty. Much of the communication is in the form of questions often directed to the leader, with very few exchanges between the members. Dainow and Bailey (1989) describe this as the group saying, 'What shall we do?'

Storming

The group is concerned with the struggles of the work and the examination of the conflicts, such as pairing, rebellion against the leader and emotional resistance to the task, as well as the interpersonal skills and interactions of group members. Dainow and Bailey (1989) describe this as, 'It can't be done' or 'I won't do it.'

Norming

The group is working together and becoming cohesive. Members feel free to expose their professional encounters without fear. An honesty of practice is established, where there is mutual support. The communications are now between members whose views and feelings are respected. Dainow and Bailey (1989) say, 'At this point the group is approaching the task with the feeling of we can do it.'

Norming is well illustrated in the above description of the work of a group of midwives; although there was a hiccough for one of the midwives, others went on to share an honesty of practice where views and feelings were respected for both patients and members of the group.

Performing

The group is now able to focus on the task. There is a flexibility of thinking and an acceptance that there may be no answers or solutions. Real listening is taking place and insights are shared with patients to gain some understanding of the anxiety. The insights of the other group members are reflected upon and action research begins. Dainow and Bailey (1989) describe the feeling here as, 'We are doing it.'

DISSOLVING THE GROUP

One aspect not previously discussed is that of ending a group. The leader will need to prepare for the dissolving of any group even if it has only met for a short time. Levine (1979) refers to this last phase as the 'termination phase', in describing the dissolution of a group or similar events. Here, if the effects are sufficiently disruptive, the group will regress to dependency or to the Forming stage (usually only a brief interlude). There may be an opportunity for reflection within the group on previous encounters where loss and grieving have been part of the story. Discussions have usually revealed how distressing it is when farewells have not been said, as happens with a sudden death. The leader is able to recall these cases and draw attention to this phase and the behaviour of the group. Saying good-bye is always important, and is an important part of the study in a psychosexual group. The leader is responsible for overseeing the parting of the group members, the evaluation of the seminars and the assessments of the group members. The group very often takes the responsibility for more informal farewells.

LEADERSHIP SKILLS

The aim of the leader is to help students develop skills for psychosexual awareness and the care of patients' sexual lives. The leader needs to have a multi-faceted approach in this coaching role and the following thoughts may be helpful when leading the seminar groups.

Achieve a flexible approach

Each person has an individual style and their own skills as a leader. The approach offered will depend on the attitude of the leader, which then determines the atmosphere. The leader has to be open-minded, creating a friendly and emotionally secure atmosphere that gives permission for practitioners to present their encounters for study and discussion. Leadership skills are developed in a unique way. An advantage of being a member of a Balint psychosexual group before becoming a leader is that there is the opportunity to watch a leadership technique. The leader should not be seen as directing, telling, prescribing or giving opinions. There is a temptation for the leader to revert to old, well tried, didactic methods of training when things are difficult, to cut corners to save time, but this is to be avoided. Experienced leaders agree that the smaller the group, the greater the temptation to instruct or tell.

The leader can be tempted to join in the discussion because they fear there will not be enough discussion from the members, therefore they start to offer their opinions and resolutions for the presented problems. Under such circumstances, their role changes from one of a coach to a didactic teacher.

The group members will always observe the leader for the individual professional and personal skills of behaviour and this includes the courtesy and respect shown to members of the group. These observations act as a philosophy of this training method, which in turn acts as a model for the development of skills for communicating with patients.

Attention to each student's needs

The leader should listen to each student, remembering particularly the unease of people who are just starting to talk about sex. Each student comes with their own experiences and skills. Indeed, some students come with many years of clinical practice. Unfortunately few come with any confidence in caring for psychosexual issues. Thus the leader's very ease and fluency in discussing sexual matters may inhibit the students. The leader, at the same time, needs to provide a model of acquired confidence to enable the practitioners to talk without inhibition. Changes of practice will need to take place to develop new skills of listening, responding and understanding the anxieties presented to practitioners. Old practices and ways of thinking have to make way for these new skills. For experienced practitioners this can be a difficult task. Each student is an individual and each will have a different way of dealing with the changes that have to be made within themselves. In order for lasting development to take place the process of change cannot be hurried by impatience. If there is pressure to do better, either from the individual practitioner or the leader, the member is much more likely to leave the group.

The low attrition rates from the students on the ENB 985 (Olive Hayden School of Midwifery 1989–1990) show evidence of this, where the mutual selection day provided knowledge of the expectations of the course, and awareness of the changes in practice and attitude that might be required (Randall 1992).

Actively involve the students

Presentations

It is important for group members to feel no pressure to present encounters; presentations are to be sought rather than demanded. The leader may ask the group, 'Who would like to present today?' There may be hesitation but there is rarely no response and usually two or three members say they have an encounter. Despite the preparedness to present, members can be inhibited by false modesty and deferential behaviour. The leader may then be required to choose, by asking one practitioner to start.

The presentation is made without notes and the group is discouraged from interrupting the story. It is not an uncommon for a student to produce a notebook in the first seminar but they can be politely asked to put it under the chair while the leader encourages the group to listen closely. The account or event is then recounted.

The presentation becomes the clinical event to be studied: the feelings, the behaviour between the two, the defences that were used, as well as the effect the patient had on the practitioner and the care that was given or offered (Chapter 2).

The leader initially may have to set an example for the presentation by reminding members to describe the following points:

◆ The setting, e.g. ward, clinic, home.
◆ How many people, e.g. single, couples, children, around?

◆ What the patient looked like, e.g. appearance, dress, hair, nails.
◆ The patient's manner, e.g. friendly, angry, unhelpful.
◆ Why was the problem presented at that time? Did the patient come out directly with the anxiety or did they wait until the end? Did the practitioner make the enquiry which revealed the anxiety?
◆ Is the presentation a suitable problem for the group to discuss? (Remember the focus is on patients' sexual lives.)
◆ How did the patient behave? Did they weep or cry? What feelings were felt by the practitioner, e.g. anger, sadness, excitement, guilt?
◆ What are the feelings the group are hearing and can identify in this practitioner–patient relationship?

The practitioner should paint a picture of the patient rather than a factual history of health or illness. Practitioners well trained in history-taking, often find this difficult at the beginning but it is surprising how quickly the group grasp what information is required and the appropriate presentation for the study of an encounter. A pattern of reporting emerges. Descriptions can leave vivid memories for the group, as in the description of a woman who arrived in the clinic wearing a bright red coat and long, beautifully manicured nails which were exactly the same colour as her coat! This description from the practitioner also set an example to the group and showed the importance of accurate observation to inform the discussion that follows.

Practitioners do observe very well but they rarely have the opportunity to report these observations and, for some, observation may even be considered to be trivial and of little clinical significance. In psychosexual work, observations provide helpful clues to anxiety and the care that may be required. During the presentation the group are usually listening intently, with the knowledge that there will be plenty of time for discussion when it is finished. Occasionally the story is too long and complicated, and the leader may choose a suitable moment at which to stop the presentation and allow the discussion to begin.

Discussions

There is no obligation for the members to comment. Students sometimes say very little but the leader will soon detect those who are listening and involved. Occasionally the leader may notice the whole group seems inattentive while they are also finding it difficult to maintain interest. The leader can then ask the group to study the case and explore this feeling of boredom, to gain some insight into the relationship between patient and practitioner. The study will almost always reveal the patient's own boredom as the root cause of the problem. Initially, members of the group will look at and directly address their accounts, questions and remarks to the leader, as well as the questions and remarks that follow. The leader has to ensure the encounters are addressed to the whole group. To encourage this, avoid eye contact. Looking down to the floor can help. In the discussion the aim is to enable general discussion from member to member, around and across the circle.

A silence in the group is often unbearable and cannot be tolerated by some. This can be an indication to the leader of how practitioners deal with silence in their work. Comments that are made, often off the cuff with no real thought or understanding behind them, can become an escape from the difficult feelings aroused by this situation. The leader can then highlight the situation to indicate how difficult it can be to tolerate not knowing. As the group progresses, the silence is tolerated and the leader may choose to break the silence to gain some insight into it by asking each member what they are feeling. Often only thoughts will be offered, but the leader has to remember that it is the practitioner–patient feelings which give a clue about the silence in relation to the encounter.

When there is a 'busy' group, there may be too much talking, sometimes evoked by the encounter or a remark from a member. Under these circumstances, members are usually not listening to each other; the leader should encourage only one person to speak at a time.

During the discussion, the leader should aim to be the last to speak or comment about the encounter. The group has to be allowed to do the work, otherwise groups will abandon the work task. If they start to wander, the leader *always* needs to remember to take the discussion back to the encounter and the study of the practitioner–patient relationship (Box 15.2).

The patient may appear to be rude and unfriendly; there is usually a reason for this. Sadly, many people's sexual lives are upset and sometimes ruined by hidden anger. It can be so much easier to work with someone who is receptive and friendly than someone who is unfriendly and angry. The leader will need to allow the group to recognise the importance of any feelings, however pain-

---

Box 15.2 Questions the leader can ask the group to keep to the task and focus of work

1. Have we any ideas about the behaviour of the practitioner with the patient?
2. What sort of practitioner was the patient getting that day? (The practitioner may have had a bad day, family problems or work pressures.)
3. What feelings were around? How did the patient make the practitioner feel? Perhaps the practitioner didn't really like the patient (often permission has to be given, preferably from within the group, that one cannot hope to or need not like everyone).

ful, as an insight into the anxiety. Once there is an insight, sharing the feeling with the patient can become a therapeutic event.

1. What defences are being used by the patient and the practitioner during the encounter?

2. What did this practitioner find difficult and what was she anxious about?

Permit freedom of thought

To permit freedom of thought the arrangements for privacy and confidentiality will have to be discussed and it is the responsibility of the leader to maintain and agree the rules with the group. The leader will need to establish that the group is a private meeting and that there are to be no interruptions. Recently, mobile equipment such as phones have intruded and a request to turn these off should be made. Confidentiality is not just about keeping secrets but it is also about the trust within the group, and having the confidence that group members will not break the agreement. Some group members may know each other outside the group in a personal capacity but the leader should ensure that any comments made between them should be confined to what they know of each other within the group. Occasionally practitioners will have patients in common and even share joint care. However, the leader ensures the study and discussion is only about the presented encounter and the relevant practitioner and patient.

The leader should maintain confidentiality about her personal life. This enables the work of the group to take place in a professional setting and without the intrusion of the members knowing about the leader's personal life.

To allow the group freedom of thought it is essential the leader holds back and refrains from intervening and making comments too early. The group members require time to listen, think and then be verbally responsive. The practitioners slowly learn that rarely is there any great revelation about the encounter but, like a jigsaw, the pieces begin to fit as discussion progresses. The leader is also listening and internally gaining insight without making an intervention at this point, however powerful the temptation to jump in and provide an understanding. The leader requires self-control. A premature interjection stops the group members from making their own discoveries and the benefits of the group's work accrue only to the leader. Each group produces its own theory and research from the presented encounters (Chapter 16).

Balance challenge and support

The leader has to bear in mind the need to keep a professional distance and at the same time offer support to the group and the individual. Initially, group members are always anxious to find the answers and solutions and therefore tend to become dependent upon the leader. One of the challenges for the leader is to get the group to accept the difficult concept of allowing anxieties and distress to go unanswered, and to recognise that there can sometimes be no solutions. Once this concept is understood, it can become a release for the practitioners from a previous constriction in their practice.

The evidence of the support offered is the containment of the group by the leader. Unless the group feels safe it will not express the trust that is essential for the growth of a group. Wright (1989) writes, 'Even if the group does move into later development stages, unless it is "contained" it will only be able to work at a fairly shallow level.'

Challenges come from group members and the leader will need to watch for destructive challenges that are undermining, humiliating and hurtful. Destructive challenges often cause feelings of anger and frustration in the leader. Anger and frustration may however be a reflection of the patient's experience. It is therefore important to study the practitioner–patient relationship to clarify why the practitioner feels as she does.

Allow students to give and receive a critique of the skill that is being acquired

As the group works together the leader will begin to notice a cohesiveness and a feeling of trust which allows for the giving and receiving of a critique. Practitioners do want to learn new skills and this hunger to learn can create dynamic forces helping both their own development and the development of others. Eventually, practitioners become more at ease with the clinical presentations, and more aware and excited by the findings. They are then able to recognise good work and offer praise. Ramprogus (1988) writes that 'A great advantage of group work with experienced nurses it seems to me, lies in its earthiness, realism and absence of pretensions.' The reflective process after the seminar will often reinforce both positive and negative comments.

Listen

The leader's ability to listen is vital for the life of a Balint seminar, and is multi-layered and demanding, just as it is for practitioners when listening to patients. It is important to understand that there may be unconscious meanings being expressed behind the overt or covert presentations.

The leader listens to:

◆ the presentation
◆ the story as it emerges

- ◆ the dialogue between patient and practitioner
- ◆ the interventions that are made by the practitioner and the patient
- ◆ the effect of the interventions if they were used
  - – were they thoughtful rather than impulsive
  - – did the practitioner think about the interventions that were not used
- ◆ the assumptions and reassurances that are made and given.

The non-verbal observations of the group members are also important. Are members:

- ◆ going to sleep
- ◆ sitting on the edges of the chairs
- ◆ showing emotion, moist eyes, upset or even distressed
- ◆ laughing, perhaps a sign of embarrassment.

In the discussion the leader has to listen to everyone; observing, as well as listening to, the practitioners' interventions and noting the group reaction. Do the group listen to some people and seem to ignore others? The leader may notice the characteristic defences of individual practitioners, e.g. they may always make a referral. Do they have any insight into their behaviour? If they make a genital examination is it treated as a therapeutic event or is it performed as a routine skill without much thought or feeling?

Many practitioners will need coaching in new ways of listening. Most practitioners are good at listening but to make the responses meaningful they also have to listen to the various layers of conversation. There may be a resistance to listening when the work is difficult for practitioners, but leaders cannot afford to avoid listening. Leaders sometimes have to tolerate periods in a seminar when they feel ignorant and helpless, and Casement (1985) writes, 'In this sense students are privileged, they have a licence not to know.' In a Balint seminar, the leader does not have to be all-knowing either and the discovery that the leader is willing and open to learning from members of the group allows for trust to develop. During the discussion the leader is then in a position to encourage critical analysis.

Patrick Casement (1985) describes, in relation to his work as a psychotherapist, how he deals with some of the pitfalls in his everyday work by 'formally developing a process of internal supervision, analysing from the patient's perspective what I think is happening'. Leaders may find using this idea of internal supervision useful to keep an eye on their leadership skills. It preserves an element of not knowing and listening for fresh understanding, even tolerating periods in a seminar of feeling incompetent and a willingness to wait until something genuinely meaningful begins to emerge in the discussion. This can also offer a role model to practitioners helping them to develop communication skills and the art of real listening.

Be caring, enthusiastic, use humour appropriately

The personality of individual leaders will be the key here. Some practitioners come to the seminar feeling uncared for in their professional work, but it is important that the leader does not allow complaints about colleagues to be discussed; the psychosexual care of the patient is the focus. The presentations will often reveal that patients feel uncared for as well.

Leaders notice that, after attending seminars and on reflection, the practitioners will often have the confidence to deal with a problem at work themselves. Common examples of these are interruptions in a consultation, a knock on the door or a request to answer the telephone. Personal caring in the seminar is not the role of the leader. If it is explained at the beginning of training that the seminar is not a therapeutic group for the personal problems of the practitioners, it rarely presents a problem. Leaders of groups have noticed that if there are some personal problems for a member of the group, it is others in the group who will often offer support and empathy. There may be changing personal circumstances for a group member but it only becomes the responsibility of the leader to make an intervention if it affects the work of the individual or the group (Chapter 6).

The leader will have to be enthusiastic, but not over-enthusiastic, to avoid Lawler's (1991) statement: 'People who have an interest in sexuality are regarded with suspicion and scepticism.' Respect for the subject itself is essential to maintain dignity and a professional role as a leader in this field.

Psychosexual awareness and care often seems to have the mantle of being very serious work. Tutor colleagues will comment with surprise, 'You do seem to have fun in your seminar.' Grigg (1997) suggests: 'Adding the proposition "Having fun is allowed!" to the ground rules helps participants to relax and to feel more comfortable.' The sexual lives of some patients can be exciting and even amusing and as long as the humour is not cruel or destructive in the group, it can throw light on the encounter that is being discussed. Laughter can be used as a way of saying to a member, 'Oh not again' in relation to an incident which has been heard before in the group. Laughter can always be studied in the patient encounters.

Allow time to practice and for reflection

All practitioners and educators have enormous pressures on them to develop and it is often seen as a race against time for this development to take place. The Balint seminar can be used as quality time for the practitioners to learn. There is much written about the need for offering quality care for the patients, but practitioners need this time as well. Human sexuality is often difficult to discuss, full of emotions and can even be controversial. Leaders always have to remember this when coaching for psychosexual awareness and care. Practitioners have to 'make room' for new learning. For some practitioners, it may take time even to make a start and the leader needs to establish an atmosphere where the practitioners can take advantage of not having the pressure to perform.

If this freedom of time and atmosphere is allowed, then the practitioners can free themselves to have 'the courage of one's own stupidity' (Balint 1964). Stupidity is also the unknown – practitioners do not have to know the answers.

Practitioners should feel free to be themselves, they do not need to act or make pretences. They can then use all their past experiences and newly acquired skills without inhibition with their patients. At the same time they learn and are able to tolerate the unknown and searching critique from within the group. The leader may have to show there is no correct or incorrect way of working but there is always new learning.

The use of reflection on the discussion about caring for patients' sexual lives is vital to a lasting change in practice. Leaders of groups have observed how easy it is for members to slip back into old ways and fail to use these new skills. Practitioners can continue to feel uncomfortable and a failure in some encounters, but with other presentations the leader and the group will recognise the development of new skills, often expressing admiration for the change that is taking place in the individual practitioner.

TRAINING AND SUPPORT FOR THE LEADER

The task of a leaders' group is to offer training in coaching and leadership skills. Without the support of a training group, the new leader especially, may start to become deskilled and disillusioned with the experience.

The leader needs to have the training and supervision to lead a group just as much as the practitioner does to develop new skills. It has to be an ongoing process. Leaders make mistakes and need exploration, with skilled help, to understand what was happening in the group.

The focus in a leaders' seminar is leading a group. The presentations are from the leaders and are the stories of their group and their experiences as leaders. It is not about the clinical presentations of the group, unless they throw some light on the behaviour of the leader and the work of the group. Without this support it is easy to slip into didactic ways of teaching. The presented material is often painful and can obstruct the leader's ability to stand back, to think and understand how the group is behaving in the here and now.

The leader of such a Balint seminar is offering supervision of the leaders' practice; experiential training that is a mirror of the practitioner group but with the focus of leading a group. For some leaders it may not be possible to attend a group or there may not be a trainer who is familiar with the work in

Case study 15.3

An experienced leader was asked to integrate some seminars into a short course on sexuality. The first course went well and had a positive evaluation with early learning of psychosexual awareness skills and an enthusiasm for the seminar training. But the second course was a different story. The managers of the course appeared not to value her work with the group, which seemed to be reflected by the students' attitudes and anxieties. No regular attendance, the presentations were complicated and difficult with the group expecting answers from the leader. On evaluation the leader learnt that some of the members had been coerced into attending.

In a leaders' seminar, this situation was discussed and the leader said she felt a destruction of her skills, she felt she would never lead a seminar again. The group studied the effect of the managerial situation on the group and the leader. It appeared it was difficult for the students to attend; there was very little encouragement for the leader from management and not much interest in the subject from some of the group. With an angry group and leader, the atmosphere was wrong to develop new skills in psychosexual awareness, with the result that little work was achieved. For the leader, without the supervision of the seminar, she admitted she would probably have given up. She continues to lead seminars as a result of the understanding she gained from the supervision of other leaders.

a Balint seminar in the locality, in which case it is recommended that telephone supervision is arranged with an experienced leader through the Association of Psychosexual Nursing.

Where a tutor or manager has never attended a seminar and feels they would like to try this approach it would be advisable to attend a workshop on Balint leadership skills. Suggestions for the organisation of a leaders workshop are outlined in Chapter 13.

REFERENCES

Balint M 1964 The doctor, his patient and the illness. Pitman Medical, London
Berne E 1964 Games people play. Penguin, New York
Bion W 1961 Experiences in groups. Tavistock, London
Casement P 1985 On learning from the patient. Tavistock, London
Dainow S, Bailey C 1989 Developing skills with people: training for person to person client contact. Wiley, Oxford
Dewey J 1974 John Dewey on education: selected writings, Archambault R D (ed) University of Chicago Press, Chicago
Erikson E 1965 Childhood and society. Penguin, London
Griffiths P, Leach G 1998 Psychosocial nursing: a model learnt from experience. In: Barnes E, Griffiths P, Ord J, Wells D (eds) Face to face with distress. Butterworth Heinemann, Oxford

Grigg E 1997 Guidelines for teaching about sexuality. Nurse Education Today 17: 62–66
Lawler J 1991 Behind the screens: nursing somology and the problem of the body. Churchill Livingstone, Melbourne
Levine B 1979 Group psychotherapy: practice and development. Prentice Hall, New York
Main T 1989 Training for the acquisition of knowledge or the development of skill? In: Johns J (ed) The ailment and other psychoanalytic essays. Free Association Books, London
Ramprogus V 1988 Groupwork in continuing nurse education: Senior Nurse 8(11): 18–20
Randall E 1992 Preparation for psychosexual nursing. Results of a survey of the ENB course 985 at the Olive Haydon School of Midwifery–Lewisham Hospital. Goldsmiths' College, London
Schon D 1987 Educating the reflective practitioner. Jossey Bass, London
Smith P 1992 The emotional labour of nursing: how nurses care. Macmillan, London
Tuckman B 1965 Developmental sequence in small groups. Psychological Bulletin 63: 384–399
Wright H 1989 Groupwork: perspectives and practice. Scutari, London

16

Other ways of training with a Balint approach

Jane Selby

KEY ISSUES

◆ Workshops
◆ Integrating Balint seminars into long or short courses
◆ Reading seminars

INTRODUCTION

In this chapter other ways of training using a Balint approach are discussed. The approach has been used extensively in workshops and it is also suitable for seminars which form a integral part of short or long courses. Reading seminars can be a useful adjunct to Balint seminars. Here the leader provides questions on a chosen article or chapter so that students can arrive prepared to discuss examples of practice which relate to the reading.

WORKSHOPS

Many sensitive practitioners are aware of their lack of knowledge and skills in how to respond to their patients' psychosexual needs. The financial and time constraints of today may dictate that long-term training is not available, but some educational authorities are willing and able to organise a day's training to answer the needs of practitioners. Our experience and evaluations of Balint-approach workshops show that the aim can only be one of psychosexual awareness in the first instance. During the workshop the strengths and weaknesses practitioners possess can be uncovered, and their anxieties about practice revealed. Practitioners soon realise that they are not alone with their thoughts and feelings. The workshop offers an experience of experiential learning where they are encouraged to talk about their own clinical encounters. Our experience shows there is never any lack of stories and material from the students to enrich the experience.

Organisation

The numbers for a workshop will depend on the availability of leaders. For a group of 25 practitioners it is advisable to have two leaders. The day can then be divided into small and large groups for learning. A maximum of 12 people with one leader is appropriate for the Balint seminar. Before the workshop, a programme and a short reading list of relevant books and journal articles should be prepared by those responsible for facilitating the day. Apart from a quiet room for the large group, and the possibility of a second room if there are two seminar groups, the leader requires only a flip chart, paper, felt pens and Blu-Tack™. It is important the leaders keep a short account of the day for reference. Some Health Trusts and colleges may require a written report of the day with evaluations.

Leader's task

The leader is present to maintain the focus on psychosexual awareness with the many different disciplines that may be present. Where there are two leaders, the programme is devised jointly and the work of the day is shared. Leading a whole-day workshop is an exhausting experience and it is good to have a short respite even if you do not leave the room.

Suggested aims

1. To help members of the workshop become more aware of the psychosexual needs of patients in their daily clinical practice.

2. To help members of the workshop explore their current practice in recognising and responding to patients' sexual health care.

If the workshop is being integrated into a specialist course the aims can be made more specific.

Intended learning outcomes

1. To have an awareness of the psychosexual needs of patients.
2. To have identified the skills required to listen and respond to patients.
3. To have participated in a Balint seminar.

Box 16.1 Responsibilities of the leader

◆ Acknowledge and dispel the anxiety that is present when sexuality is on the agenda, allowing for the vulnerability of the students, however experienced they may appear

◆ Focus on the aim

◆ Outline how the programme will be achieved

◆ Explain that the day will be participative

◆ Explain that no personal problems will be discussed

◆ Explain that the study will be the practitioner–patient relationship in their professional role

◆ Explain there is no role play

◆ Give a brief description of working in a seminar, explaining that they will have a chance to talk of recent patient encounters. No preparation of material is required

◆ Provide a safe and comfortable working atmosphere

◆ Maintain strict time-keeping

◆ Make introductions that permit the above to be achieved

◆ Outline the boundaries of the day.

Programme

The programme for the workshop can be devised to suit the time available and allow for flexibility in the students' learning. During the introduction, ask the participants to write down two or three things that they hope to achieve from the workshop; this may show their expectations. It also offers a chance to the leaders to be flexible and take account of the needs of the group, while maintaining the aims of the day and the focus. Maintaining the focus can be helped by asking the group to identify patients' psychosexual anxieties and the individual member's problems of working with these anxieties. The discussion that follows allows for an awareness to develop and a recognition of skills members of the group may already possess. For instance, you may ask:

1. What are the problems you have in responding to your patients' sexual needs?

2. Identify the sexual health needs and anxieties of the patients that you meet.

These questions allow students to think for themselves individually or in small groups and the answers are recorded for discussion and clarification. The leader can then invite students to illustrate the points from their clinical practice, producing many different objective and subjective sensitivities and the chance for the leader to allow freedom of thought from the group.

A listening exercise can also be useful, as one of the most important skills in psychosexual work is the art of listening. After a disciplined listening exercise even experienced students are surprised at themselves as they recognise their temptations to interrupt, offer thoughts and ideas and then realise they may be doing this in their everyday practice.

A Balint seminar of 1.5–2 hours is a useful way of allowing members of the group to present encounters verbatim with no preparation, the only stipulation being that it is a recent psychosexual encounter with a patient. The discussion is a valuable time for reflection on their practice. Often the leader and group show that the work is valued and respected, which gives the presenter courage to begin to think about changes they might consider in their practice.

Evaluation

The students are encouraged to write and express their feelings of the day:

1. Describe your experience of the workshop.
2. What new or revised learning have you experienced today?
3. Do you have any ideas for change in addressing the sexual health needs of your patients?
4. Any other comments.

At the end of a workshop there are usually some who have found this approach particularly valuable and who feel they would like to continue developing their awareness and skills in Balint seminars. These people, together with a leader, may be the stimulus for a new group to form in the locality.

INTEGRATING BALINT SEMINAR TRAINING INTO SHORT OR LONG COURSES

The seminar approach can be integrated into any training where the patient's emotional and psychosexual care is part of the curriculum. There is no reason this method should not be open to practitioners in many different specialties. The learning also covers the art of communication for developing and increasing the sensitive skills that all practitioners require. Post-basic students find that, with more clinical responsibilities, they often lack the skills to offer the holistic care they would wish, especially where there is little time or space in a busy working environment. A seminar is an ideal time to reflect and think about new approaches with patients, and to consider ways of helping patients' sexual lives by studying the practitioner–patient relationship in the presented encounters (Chapter 14). Benner (1984) writes, 'nurses at the proficient and expert levels can benefit from exchanges, clinical case studies, and opportunities to conduct and participate in research on clinical problems'. All these are available when attending a Balint seminar training.

Suggested framework

All tutors who are participating in the course need to be fully briefed and to understand the philosophy of the training, otherwise conflicting views may prove confusing for everyone. It is important for tutors to consider how the psychosexual work links with the rest of the teaching. Discussions about holistic care and psychosexual care both amongst the tutors and with students can help psychosexual work to be seen as an important aspect of care rather than something separate. Integration can then be part of the total experience in a variety of learning experiences for the practitioners and tutors: in lectures, other group activities, written assignments, reading seminars and in the clinical workplace.

Aim of training

The aim is to develop awareness and skills to work with patients who have sexual health care needs in the course of practitioners' everyday clinical practice.

Workshop in the introductory block

During an introductory study block it is advisable to have 1 day organised as a psychosexual workshop devoted to sharing the anxieties and problems that patients may experience. When practitioners talk about their patient concerns, with careful coaching they can also perceive their own anxieties and their own skills. As these anxieties and skills are identified each practitioner may be able to make a list of their own needs for skill development and change. This workshop sets the scene for the experiential learning that will take place in the following seminars.

Seminar training

There should be about six seminars of 1.5–2 hours in length in a short course (up to 6 months) – at least one a month. The time is often dictated by the material that has to be taught but this number of seminars allows for a continuous process of learning in a busy programme of theory and clinical work. Seminars can be held during study days or block periods. The seminars with a leader involve an in-depth study of the practitioner–patient relationship based on the student presentations of recent clinical encounters (Chapter 14). Where the course is longer than 6 months, more seminars can be integrated to continue training over the full period of the course.

Learning outcomes

These outcomes are more likely to be achieved when there is sharing of the experiences and participation by all the group members. The leader is the coach, and offers a model to the practitioners of listening and trying to understand the presented encounter.

It is recommended that other theoretical aspects of emotional care which may affect the patient should be studied in conjunction with the seminars, e.g. in lectures, group discussions, individual presentations or reading seminars. There is then an opportunity for a more generalised study of the possible emotional experiences that may occur, e.g. loss (Section 2).

Written assignments

As part of the training, written assignments are required; every practitioner writes up an account of the seminar. A brief account of each case history is recorded but the account concentrates on the group's discussion, with the reflections noted for future practice. The emphasis in the learning is through the sharing and participation of all members of the group.

Box 16.2 Learning outcomes

◆ Awareness of how the patient presents

◆ Insight into what happened in the here and now

◆ Develop an understanding of feelings – both the practitioners' and patients'

◆ Explore what the practitioner finds difficult

◆ Understand what the patient finds difficult

◆ Understand how the practitioner works with different patients

◆ Develop skills of listening, responding and reflecting to have an increased understanding of the sexual needs of patients.

The resumé of the seminar focusses on the following aspects:

1. The interaction of the practitioner and the patient. How did this patient make the practitioner feel? What happened in the here and now?
2. What did the practitioner find difficult/was anxious about?
3. What did the patient find difficult/was anxious about?
4. What, if any, defences did the practitioner use?
5. Any new insights gained.
6. Anything that impressed the practitioner as others shared their thoughts and feelings.
7. What was the effect of the intervention?

Evaluation

The overall evaluation of a course integrating a workshop and seminars (Bell et al 1997) was recorded as:

◆ Active listening, responding, reflecting and interpreting without making assumptions
◆ Focussing on feelings; staying with the clients' distress to understand their anxiety, rather than just giving advice or reassurance
◆ Understanding each anxiety in its uniqueness and the particular meaning for each patient.

In one workshop and six seminars there cannot be the same development as in a longer series of seminars. But where previously there had been little attention to the patients' sexual lives, after even this short training, the group members and tutors noticed there was nearly always a marked and often exciting improvement in their skills of addressing patients' sexual needs. Some practitioners become aware that these changes require further training and supervision of practice. They can then join or start new seminars where this can be continued and becomes a useful method of supervision of practice.

READING SEMINARS

Reading seminars can be organised to support the understanding of the relationship of texts to practice. These are discussion seminars and each is based on a specific journal article or chapter from a book. Students attending Balint seminars are expected to read widely, both from the suggested texts and according to their own interests. It is useful in a reading seminar to make a detailed analysis and evaluation of a few texts. The aim is to demonstrate the approach to reading which can render as much value from the texts as possible in relation to patients' care. To achieve this, the seminar leader usually provides a series of questions related to the text to help the students:

1. Identify the issues in the text
2. Consider the implications for the students' practice
3. Relate the ideas from 1 & 2 to other learning (practical and theoretical).

As the course progresses the students will take increasing responsibility to generate their own questions in order to interrogate the text and make links with both practice and earlier learning. The leader of a reading seminar does not have to have participated or been the leader of a Balint seminar, but they should be familiar with the philosophy behind any course to make the text relevant to the students' clinical practice.

When the course is about a specific specialty the texts can be chosen to highlight particular theories, research and emotional care that is involved. Provocative texts can be a challenge as well as a stimulus to a group where they are encouraged to have freedom of thought. When the group is studying patients' emotional care, Chapter 2, 'Illness, distress and neglect' in Keith Nichols' (1993) book *Psychological Care in Physical Illness* offers an excellent text for a first reading seminar with any group of practitioners. In *this* book, Section 2 offers a foundation for understanding lifestyles and emotional development in both health and illness.

CONCLUSION

Despite the ever-present budgetary constraints within the Health Service, these approaches are considered by many to be cost efferctive. A well-trained practitioner is a more efficient practitioner and, as discussed, a Balint approach can fit into several formats. Attending a Balint seminar just once can be an illuminating experience which increases the practitioner's confidence and may also encourage her to seek further training.

REFERENCES

Bell J, Rutter M, Selby J, Ward M 1997 Nurse-led family planning. Practice Nurse 14(4): 265–267
Benner P 1984 From novice to expert: excellence and power in clinical nursing practice. Addison Wesley, Menlo Park, CA
Nichols K 1993 Psychological care in physical illness, 2nd edn. Chapman & Hall, London

17

Reflective practices and action research in Balint seminars

Jane Selby

KEY ISSUES

- ◆ Reflective practices
- ◆ Reflection in Balint seminars
- ◆ Knowing and unknowing
- ◆ Clinical supervision
- ◆ Reflective diaries and written accounts of seminars
- ◆ Action research

INTRODUCTION

In this chapter Balint seminars are discussed as a method of reflection, where health professionals can study their interactions with patients. The Balint approach is compared with other methods of reflection and the differences are highlighted. Balint seminars are also discussed as a method of supervision where the coaching is offered by the leader of the group. The importance of students writing accounts of their own practice and the seminars is considered. The rigorous description and analysis both in discussion and in written records supports the idea of Balint seminars as action research.

REFLECTIVE PRACTICES

Health care professionals are being encouraged to use reflection for the development of their practice (Benner 1984, UKCC 1995, 1996, Johns 1995). Since the Balint approach is a particular way of helping practitioners to develop skills through reflection, it is important to consider the similarities and differences to be found between this (Balint) approach and other methods of reflection. The writings of Schon (1984, 1987) and Benner (1984) have been influential in health care, and so the salient features of these will be discussed and compared with those of a Balint approach.

Limits of technical rationality

Schon (1983) has pointed out that much professional education is based on an assumption that clients' problems can be solved through the use of appropriate knowledge, but this approach often fails. It might work if clients' problems were clear, logical and presented as tidy questions. However, most problems, Schon (1983) argues, are not well formed, but are indeterminate and messy. Therefore often the professional's first job is to formulate the appropriate questions. Readers may recognise this situation: although some patients arrive with a specific problem or request, frequently the first task is to clarify the patient's concern. It is important that the patient and practitioner work on this clarification together. Schon's idea that the professional, although skilled and knowledgeable, still works from ignorance in any new situation fits well with the Balint approach.

Discovery of theory

When questions have been formulated the answers are, Schon (1983) argues, not necessarily available in the professional's knowledge. Instead the professional needs to discover the answers. This means that theory is not something to be applied, but something to be discovered. Fish & Purr (1991) in a report to the ENB noted that this idea of Schon's could be revolutionary in nurse education.

Making 'tacit knowledge' visible

Although there is often a need to form questions and discover theory (Schon 1983), that does not mean that professionals lack knowledge and skills. Their knowledge and skills are, however, often 'tacit' – embedded in practice. Reflection is a valuable method for putting these into words, and making them visible (Benner 1984). Balint seminars are used in this way (Clifford 1998).

Reflection in and on action

Schon (1983) distinguishes between reflection *in* action and reflection *on* action, a valuable distinction that is also observed in Balint seminars (Clifford 1998).

Reflection *in* action refers to the rapid appraisal made of a situation whilst working with a patient.

Reflection *on* action is the retrospective thinking, which takes place after the clinical work, for example when presenting a practitioner–patient encounter for group discussion.

The cyclical process can be observed in seminars as new skills are noted and recorded.

The reflections can be undertaken by the practitioner alone or on a one-to-one basis, but there are benefits in a group:

1. The group members are willing to listen and be supportive to each other.

2. The 'fresh unrehearsed story' (de Lambert 1998) of a recent experience may reveal important thoughts and feelings, but the person giving the account may be unaware of these. Frequently it is in the telling of the story that awareness is raised, particularly when group members point out what they have understood from listening.

3. In these seminars the clear focus and the context in which it is practised permit open observations not only of personal development but also professional performance for evaluation.

Development of reflection in the Balint approach

The place of feelings and thoughts

In Balint seminars the use of feelings is considered a most valuable way to understand patients' emotional lives, but thoughts cannot be excluded and indeed must be part of the skills for any practitioner. They are used as part of an interaction, helping each person to gain insight to the presented problem. Once the practitioner is aware of the feeling, can identify and name it, this helps the thinking to take place and the discussion to move forward. The thoughts to be examined could be:

◆ Why did they get so angry?
◆ How did they present the anxiety?
◆ What did I do to make them cry?
◆ Why was I left feeling so burdened?

The following questions might be asked of oneself when reflecting in action:

◆ What is happening now between us?
◆ Where do we go from here?
◆ Do I want to hear any more?

Like a kaleidoscope, ever changing and often moving too fast, the distress may be too great and then the thoughts are lost, the moment has passed and the patient may have been left with the distress. But the great advantage for the practitioner is that the encounter can be presented in the seminar for reflection *on* action.

For many who write about reflections, feelings are not included or are only discussed as another approach to thinking about problems. In the Balint seminars, the awareness of feelings offers another dimension to understanding patients. What patients feel is, as for all of us, related to what matters in life, our values, beliefs and what is precious, difficult or painful. In people's sexual lives, relationships and memories are often of special concern. When these are considered in the Balint seminar and are shown to be central to what matters most, then the subjective assessment and emotional intervention has its place. Dealing with emotions is not easy but most practitioners can remember feeling effective and satisfied with an encounter where they remember the use of emotions. The Balint seminar can both assess and inform practice to help practitioners to develop such work and not leave it to intuition or chance.

The following encounter between a physiotherapist and her client (see case study) shows some of the reflective practices that were taking place.

Case study 17.1

The young woman, Ann, fair-haired and attractive, arrived to see the physiotherapist with two young vocal children. Ann had been referred by her GP feeling sore and with stress incontinence, with a request for some exercises and ultrasound treatment. The second baby had been a forceps delivery and the midwife had commented after the birth, 'This poor girl has been really knocked about'. She had had some immediate treatment for soft tissue injury prior to going home and was now 4 months post-delivery. The physiotherapist enquired about her symptoms and the following dialogue took place:

Physiotherapist: *Your symptoms don't seem too bad but what does it feel like for you?*

Ann: *I just feel a mess, that's all.*

Physiotherapist: *You don't look it, so I wonder what is troubling you?*

Ann: *I've lost interest in everything except the children, I just feel tired all the time. I should be so happy, I've got everything going for me.*

Physiotherapist: *How about your sex life?*

Ann: *Well ... it isn't...*

Physiotherapist: *Was it OK before the children?*
Ann: *Yes, fine right up to this baby.*
Physiotherapist: *What are we going to do with you!* (they laughed together)
Ann: *My doctor looked down below and everything is healed, he said.*
I seem to have nothing to show for the troubles I am having.
Physiotherapist: *It is not a happy situation.* (the children were very restive)
Ann: *It all feels sort of wrong there and not a bit like I felt before she*
was born.
Physiotherapist: *How would it be if you came back without the children and we*
will have another look at the problem and if necessary treat you?
Ann: *Yes, please, I do want to feel right again.* (the children were
roaring and she left)

This is a familiar story, heard by many practitioners as they see patients in their everyday practice, where a sexual life has been disrupted for a healthy woman in the course of a natural event. Similar disruptions may occur with or following illness. This physiotherapist was experienced in her field but was also able to reflect *in* action as she worked with her patient. It seemed there was more to the problem than the orginal presentation suggested, but there was no space for discussion with the patient's restive children present. The practitioner and patient needed privacy to discuss this intimate situation.

This encounter was brought to a seminar where the reflection *on* action took place. The discussion by the members of the group brought to light the relationship of Ann and the physiotherapist, which was open, honest and with feelings acknowledged. The use of the word 'we' implied that they accepted the work was between them both. There was no need of immediate treatment but the emotional healing had perhaps begun after this particular meeting. The seminar members admired the skills of this practitioner. But they also reminded her of a previous occasion when there had been no mention of sex in a similar case. The physiotherapist laughed and said, 'I have not forgotten that seminar', nor had the group (see Fig. 17.1).

Engaging in care

When a patient's sexual life becomes disrupted or disordered by life events or illness, they often seek help. As Schon (1983) explained, however, the skills and knowledge which can help are not available in prepared packages and prescriptions. Instead both practitioner and patient need to engage – building a bridge describes this process – so that the patient's concern may be formu-

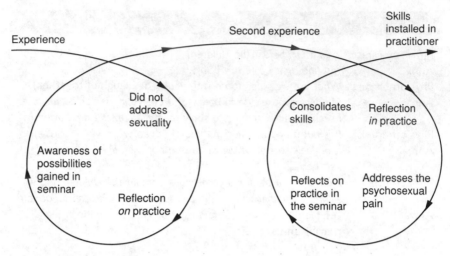

Fig. 17.1 Reflective cycles

lated (Chapter 3). Patients, like practitioners, often have tacit knowledge, i.e. they know their concerns or problems but have not yet put them into words. Benner (1984) makes the point about involvement of the practitioner being the hallmark of the expert – not always acknowledged in patient care but clearly acknowledged in Balint work. The encounter between Ann and the physiotherapist shows they engaged during their meeting, a mutual honesty and co-equality were established and the work started. Sometimes practitioners may feel they have gone too far. The seminar approach is a way of developing the required skills to enable this bridge to be built between the patient and the practitioner.

In the Balint seminars the encounters shared by the practitioners, and the subsequent discussions, usually focus on who was there, what happened and what feelings were aroused in the practitioner. The reflection is then on any insight that was achieved through the awareness of feelings at the time, afterwards, or during the seminar:

1. Does this enlighten the practitioner and the group members about the relationship formed with the patient?
2. What sort of engagement was made?
3. Did this increase the understanding of the patient?

Knowing and unknowing

The leader's role is to maintain the focus of study throughout the discussion. It is often hard to keep all the group members focussed on the encounter that has been reported. As they are reminded of similar situations there is a temptation to offer their own story but that usually only detracts from the study. A brief reflection on another situation may be helpful, particularly if it has been discussed in a previous seminar, but a new story diverts attention.

Whilst maintaining the focus on the practitioner and her experience, there are two important and apparently contradictory principles for the leader to remember. First, competent and even proficient practitioners may not recognise their own skills until they are commented on in the group, either by the members or the leader. This recognition is often adopted by the group members and becomes a valuable feature of peer support. Heath (1998) endorses this: 'Reflective practice should also be used to identify why a situation went well as this will identify the knowledge embedded in practice that will enrich nursing, enabling the practitioners to assess their professional development and, by providing understanding of actions be used to guide less experienced nurses.' Second, no matter what expertise is available, it is important to approach the work with the patient from a state of ignorance. Doreen Clifford talks of the practitioner being led and coached by the patient. Similarly the group leader, whilst possessing skills in group work, learns from the group members as they explore their clinical practice through reflection. This delicate balance between leaders and seminar members and between leading and learning is discussed in Chapters 14 and 15.

Benefits of reflective practice in Balint seminars

◆ Skilled practice which may be taken for granted is made visible, acknowledged and valued.
◆ As reflective practice is developed the seminar develops its own theory.
◆ Recounting stories and the discussions that follow allow for clarification of the encounter.
◆ The exploration of the feelings and thoughts of patients/practitioners are revealed by the unrehearsed stories.
◆ Support that is offered allows increased perceptions concerning the work.
◆ Knowing the how and why of an encounter leads to the practitioner being more flexible in approach.
◆ Knowledge sought by the practitioner is more likely to be relevant to the practice.
◆ The leader's role is crucial to the focus of study and reflection in and on practice.

CLINICAL SUPERVISION

As in reflective practice the characteristics of clinical supervision have been much debated and interpreted in many different ways. The UKCC have now stated that 'every practitioner should have access to clinical supervision' and they have laid down the criteria with suggested models of supervision (UKCC 1995). The Department of Health (1992) defined it as 'A formal process of professional support and learning which enables individual practitioners to develop knowledge and competence, assume responsibility for their own practice and enhance consumer protection for their own practice and safety of care in complex clinical situations.'

The Balint seminar certainly falls into the required criteria for supervision because the clinical supervision offered is one of support for the practitioners by other group members and the leader. The psychosexual work discussed in the group comes from their everyday clinical practice where the development of skills and evaluation take place. This is an active learning process for all participants.

Butterworth & Faugier (1998) write, 'Clinical supervision can both empower and support those in practice and must therefore be developed by and through them, as the process of clinical supervision rests on an immediate experience of learning and can only be realised by those actively working in practice.'

In Cornwall, a group of community midwives, after attending a short series of six seminars, felt that the Balint psychosexual seminar complemented their supervised practice. They then requested that these should continue; as a result funding was granted by Cornwall Healthcare Trust. They meet every two months for 2 hours and the seminars are written up by each midwife. They are also using reflective diaries to record their work with women who have undergone termination of pregnancy. They realised as a result of the presentations and discussions in the previous seminars that some of the women they were meeting when 'booking' continued to carry the emotional distress of undergoing a termination of pregnancy. At the time of writing, they have been surprised but pleased to find how many women have appreciated the opportunity to talk about the experience.

The practitioners attending the advanced seminar (Chapter 18) also find that this supervision is essential for their continuing practice. In all counselling situations it is recommended that practitioners should attend clinical supervision of their ongoing case load (British Association of Counselling).

Butterworth and Faugier (1998) suggest, 'in a profession (nursing) which embraces mentorship and supervision it is permissible to identify a number of 'ground rules.'

The following are the 'ground rules' they suggest and are relevant for supervision in a Balint seminar.

1. 'Skills should be constantly redefined and improved throughout professional life.' Working with people's sexual and emotional lives requires a constant redefining of personal and professional skills. In a seminar there is the space

and time to allow this to occur. Often practitioners find that skills can 'slip' and in the seminar they recognise the need for constant review on a regular basis.

2. 'Critical debate about practice activity is a means to professional development.' In the seminar, each presentation is open for critical debate. This debate, held in a safe environment, allows for trust and honesty of practice to be valued where practitioners can be empowered to work with their patients. This development in skills then acts as a model of sexual care in the practitioner's working environment.

3. 'Clinical supervision offers protection and accountable practice.' Each practitioner recounts a clinical event and the responsibilities that took place. This allows for accountable practice and offers protection to the patient and practitioner. The seminar can act as an assessor of these new skills for example recognizing the boundaries that are required for safe practice.

4. 'Introduction to a process of clinical supervision should begin in professional training and education, and continue thereafter as an integral part of professional development.' Balint seminars can be integrated into any professional training but their development has mainly taken place with health care professionals and they are particularly suitable for the practitioner who has gained some experience in their field. The individual strengths and weaknesses of practitioners may be exposed and their competence monitored by the group, which acts as a measure of the quality of care that is offered to patients.

5. 'Clinical supervision requires time and energy and is not an incidental event.' The commitment of those who attend the seminars is demonstrated by regular attendance. A wish to help and support their patients comes from practitioners with a determination to try not to ignore or neglect the sexual aspect of care for each patient. Time and energy, particularly emotional energy, will be required to develop these new skills, and the process of learning in a seminar is often quite slow. Clinical supervision has to be supported by a supervisor; in the Balint seminar training this will be a leader and a coach. The skills for this task are discussed under 'Leadership skills' in Chapter 15.

RELECTIVE DIARIES AND WRITTEN ACCOUNTS OF SEMINARS

Reflective diaries

Learning diaries are a way for practitioners to record events and issues. Increasingly these are being used in undergraduate programmes (Fish & Purr 1991). In Balint seminars the unrehearsed story is crucial since practitioners indicate what was experienced when close to the patient. Frequently the way the story is told shows what happened. A carefully written account may have lost or glossed over certain features. Nevertheless there are never enough seminars to hear all the narratives from all the practices, so reflective diaries are another method of expressing, at least to oneself, psychosexual encounters and the feelings aroused by these.

The midwives who meet regularly in a Balint seminar have realised that pregnant women who have had an earlier pregnancy terminated continue to think about it. Contrary to the midwives' earlier assumptions, these women have welcomed an opportunity to discuss the thoughts and feelings they are having in relation to this. Group members record all their interactions on this topic to see what benefits or problems there are, and what skills are being developed. Such careful study is an example of Schon's (1983) idea that theory is created by reflective practitioners. This approach to skill development also fits the criteria for action research (Holter & Schwartz Barcott 1993).

Written accounts of the seminars

Members of the practitioner Balint groups have always been encouraged to keep individual written accounts of the seminars they attend. These have often been informal, when the seminar is not part of a course or a module, but, in a validated training, diaries can be one of the assessment tools.

These accounts are the story of the seminar itself, i.e. the case histories are only described briefly and the discussions that follow are recorded in more detail. The group members are asked to record their own learning outcomes, which may vary from member to member. The importance of sharing the thinking and feeling is recognised as part of the learning process and normally takes place in the discussion, but sometimes things are left unsaid. When writing up the seminar, practitioners may reflect again for themselves. These reflections are very often raised at other seminars where the presentation reminds group members of past cases with similar circumstances or issues that are under discussion. The encounter between the physiotherapist and Ann was an example of this, where the physiotherapist talked about Ann's sexual life but in a previous encounter had failed to mention sex at all.

The writing does not have to be in a formal language suitable for an essay or assignment. It is often difficult to write about the feelings of a practitioner–patient relationship and the group members should not feel inhibited to record how *they* feel. The patients cannot be identified by name and if assessment is to take place then a letter of the alphabet can be subsituted to keep the encounter anonymous. These records, and the reflective practices that take place, form the theory of practice and are a natural entry into action research of the practitioners' clinical work. These can all be identified as effective tools for implementing change in their clinical practice.

ACTION RESEARCH

The original seminars set up by Dr Michael Balint were called 'research-cum-training' seminars. They were recorded by a shorthand typist, almost verbatim, and the material used for Balint's research. He wrote, 'our research was deliberately kept self-contained' (Balint 1957). Main (1974) wrote, 'the training method is investigative of the patient's and doctor's feelings during each clinical encounter. Inevitably each seminar throws up its own findings so that every seminar could be described as one of research-cum-training.'

Action research is a method of research that involves taking action to improve practice and systematically studying the effects of the action taken (Jenks 1999). Holter & Schwartz Barcott explain that 'whereas all action research is concerned with keeping theory and practice close together, in the enhancement approach the researcher raises questions about the underlying assumptions and values and involves the practitioner in critically reflecting on their practice ... Local theory emerges from reflective discussions between the researcher and the practitioners, and emerging patterns of new practice and new theoretical insights stem from the newly formed culture of practice' (Holter & Schwartz Barcott 1993). They found no examples of this approach to action research but suggested that reflective practice would fit this theoretical perspective.

Penman (1998) has described Balint seminars as a form of action research using the 'enhancement' approach:

As a member of an advanced psychosexual seminar group, and as a leader of a group, I have been experiencing not only my own but others' significant changes in clinical practice throughout the rigorous description and analysis of case encounters.

The use of the Balint model of seminars seems to run parallel to that described by Holter and Schwartz Barcott in the enhancement approach to action research. This opens the door to a research environment in which the experiences of practitioner/patient encounters can undergo critical reflection. The individual practitioner and the group of co-equals become aware of their underlying values and assumptions concerning sexual difficulties and distress. The group forms its own unique culture of practice which energises and enables the individual practitioner to acknowledge painful, difficult encounters and to analyse both success and failure. A dynamic continuum of clinical materials is brought, described and investigated to which the practitioner chooses to respond. Theory then adapts and changes, moves on with each new encounter. What is known, tried and tested is stored and held in tension with the value of 'not knowing' when faced with a patient in psychosexual pain.

*Resolution for the patient is often profound using this approach.
The practitioner's and leader's willingness to be involved in this form of
action research using the Balint methodology leads to continued significant
change and to the ongoing development of clinical practice.*

Penman (1998) expands on this action research in her article, to illustrate
that the Balint seminar provides a working model and allows the study of the
therapeutic potential of the practitioner in each individual patient encounter.
Jenks (1999) summarises action research and states:

*Action research can be an effective method for implementing change in
today's health care environment. Its major advantage is that it creates
practical solutions to everyday nursing practice problems. Because it
involves implementation and evaluation of new ideas, action research also
provides an answer to the gap between theory and practice. Action research
is a dynamic process that involves cycling among analyses, action, reflection
and evaluation. Participants in action research are active members of the
research team, participating in the planning, implementation, and
evaluation of the action taken. When used appropriately, action research
can result in lasting change that creates a more meaningful nursing
practice. (pp xx)*

This research, although not yet undertaken in a formal way, can be seen to
take place over a period of time in the Balint seminars. It is particularly evident
in the basic and advanced seminars where the members are committed to
attend for a period of time. The analyses, actions, reflections and evaluations
can all be observed and a permanent change in their everyday work is
practised and recorded by the practitioners who have trained under the Balint
approach.

CONCLUSION

This chapter has compared Balint seminars with other methods of reflection.
Whilst feelings are often noted in reflection, their significance is very specific
in Balint-style work since the practitioner's feelings often mirror those of the
patient. The chapter has discussed how Balint seminars fulfil the requirements for both supervision and action research.

REFERENCES

Balint M 1957 The doctor, his patient and the illness. Pitman Medical, London
Benner P 1984 From novice to expert. Addison Wesley, Menlo Park, CA
British Association of Counselling Code of ethics and practice for counsellors. BAC, Rugby

Butterworth T, Faugier J 1998 Clinical supervision as an emerging idea. In: Butterworth T, Faugier J, Burnard P (eds) Clinical supervision and mentorship in nursing, 2nd edn. Stanley Thomes, London

Clifford D 1998 Psychosexual awareness in everyday nursing: Nursing Standard 12(39): 42–45

de Lambert L 1998 Learning through experience. In: Barnes E, Griffiths P, Ord J, Wells D (eds) Face to face with distress. Butterworth Heinemann, Oxford

Department of Health 1992 Vision for the future. HMSO, London

Fish D, Purr D 1991 An evaluation of practice-based learning in continuing education in nursing, midwifery and health visiting. A report for the ENB. ENB, London

Heath H 1998 Reflection and patterns of knowing in nursing: Journal of Advanced Nursing 27: 1054–1059

Holter M, Schwartz Barcott D 1993 Action research: what is it? How has it been used and how can it be used in nursing. Journal of Advanced Nursing 18: 298–304

Jenks J 1999 Action research method. In: Streubert H, Carpenter D (eds) Qualitive research in nursing: advancing the humanistic imperative, 2nd edn. Lippincott, Philadelphia, 251–263

Johns C 1995 Framing learning through reflection within Carper's fundamental ways of knowing in nursing. Journal of Advanced Nursing 22: 226–234

Main T 1989 Training for the acquisition of knowledge or the development of skill? In: Johns J (ed) The ailment and other psychoanalytical essays. Free Association Books, London

Penman J 1998 Action research in the care of patients with sexual anxieties. Nursing Standard 13: 13–15, 47–50

Schon D 1983 The reflective practitioner. Basic Books, New York

Schon D 1987 Educating the reflective practitioner. Jossey Bass, London

UKCC 1995 Clinical supervision resource pack. National Health Executive, London

UKCC 1996 Position statement on clinical supervision for nursing and health visiting. UKCC, London

18

Advanced Balint seminars

Jane Selby

KEY ISSUES

- Membership of advanced seminars
- The work of the seminar
- Supervision and support
- Leadership skills
- Joining an advanced seminar
- A researcher's viewpoint

INTRODUCTION

Everyone active in psychosexual practice, seeing patients in their own right, needs the support of continuing training for supervision. One of the opportunities for practitioners is to join a Balint advanced group, with the proviso they have attended basic Balint seminars continuously for 2 years. The advanced seminar has been formed for the development of practitioners who have demonstrated their ability to learn through the Balint approach. The learning is assessed both by their work in the seminars and in writing. Written reports are made by the seminar members and at the end of a year self-evaluations show their own development. These can be used by the seminar leader for the purpose of assessment for progression into an advanced seminar.

These seminars started in 1993 and are held monthly, in London, led by members of the Association of Psychosexual Nursing. It may not be possible for some people to have this opportunity but it is important for psychosexual practitioners to continue with supervision and not to be isolated in this difficult work. The Association organises study days for the members and can also be a valuable source of information. By attending these study days the practitioners have the chance to assess their practice in the principles of Balint training by meeting other health care workers who are involved or interested in this approach. The contact can also enable practitioners to meet members who could be willing to act as mentors or supervisors. The supervision, which could take place in a meeting or by a telephone conversation, allows the practitioner to look at the psychosexual skills she is using and monitor her performance, but it cannot offer the diversity of opinions of a seminar group.

Members of the group

The following encounters are from a group which has been in existence since 1992. All the members are experienced practitioners working in a variety of nursing fields: general practice, university health clinic, family planning, counsellor in an assisted conception unit, a young person's walk-in clinic, and termination of pregnancy units. Some work as psychosexual practitioners in the National Health Service and receive direct referrals; others are expanding their practice as they continue to develop psychosexual skills as an aspect of their work, for example as practice nurses and as university health counsellors. As practitioners advance in this work, their training responsibilities increase.

Most advanced practitioners run workshops and lead regular seminars and clinical supervision sessions. The Balint approach is appropriate for all of these.

The following case study illustrates the supervisory role that one seminar member undertook to help a colleague who felt inadequate when she was asked to see a patient. She told of a meeting with a Sister who worked in a gynaecological outpatients department.

Case study 18.1

The Sister was worrying about how she would work with a woman patient she was due to see the following day. When asked about her contact with this woman so far, she described meeting her in a consultation with a doctor, where they understood the problem as one of 'non-consummation' and the doctor asked the patient to make an appointment with the Sister, to advise her on the use of vaginal dilators. The patient failed to turn up for the appointment, but the Sister phoned and encouraged her to come at another time. Now, the Sister was wondering how to work with this problem and a seemingly reluctant patient. In discussion the supervisor and Sister were able to explore what the patient might be reluctant about and how this kind of exploration might allow the Sister to think, with the

Case study 18.1 (cont'd)

patient, what sort of help was needed. It seemed likely that self-vaginal dilatation was not acceptable to the patient. The appropriate help might be discovered when they met.

With this supervision the Sister was able to move from feeling awkward about a prescriptive treatment, through thinking and feeling how to work with the reluctant patient. It seemed the Sister was already aware of the woman's negative feelings through both the non-attendance for the appointment, and the telephone conversation. If she could continue this work in the next appointment, then the exploration might discover what the patient herself might want as help for her difficulty.

Work of the advanced seminar

The struggle for further learning continues in the advanced seminar but, as one nurse comments, 'one is more willing to struggle'. The work changes and practitioners are able to work in more complex situations, but the principles of training remain the same (Chapter 14). When practitioners join the advanced seminar they could be considered as 'proficient' (Benner 1984) since the patient is recognised as a whole person. The practitioner is trying to work alongside the patient, both to understand the issue and to create a partnership that will sustain the work. Both the partnership and the work rely on the practitioner allowing herself to feel what the patient feels. Often the feelings experienced by the practitioner emanate from the patient's world. This experience can then be acknowledged at the time, or later to inform practice. An example of this could be when one hears a patient say, 'It's not normal' or 'I don't think it is normal.' The practitioner will want to explore what 'normal' means to the patient and whether normality has any use in the interpretation of the problem. The practitioner's experience usually shows it is more likely to be the patient's perspective than some rule of normal behaviour.

When the psychosexual practitioner feels confident to work alongside patients and take clinical responsibility for the care of people's sexual lives, accepting referrals from other professionals with confidence, the practitioner may move to become an 'expert' (Benner 1984). Dreyfus & Dreyfus (1977) describe the experienced performer as one who 'is no longer aware of features and rules, and his/her performance becomes fluid and flexible and highly proficient.' But when there are difficulties in the work, a psychosexual practitioner's experience alerts her to seek supervision and support, particularly beneficial when the encounters and behaviours of patients are complex and include sexual dysfunction.

The intention in the Balint approach is to offer 'brief intervention' and not long-term treatment or therapy. Under the constraints of the National Health Service our experience informs us that the provision for psychosexual appointments is limited. This constraint often requires a self-discipline of practice and a time scale for the practitioner and patient. In the work of the advanced psychosexual practitioner there may also be a greater frequency of tangible endings than is experienced by practitioners in a basic seminar.

Supervision and support

Attending the seminar reminds members of the importance of identifying the psychosexual focus, and staying with the practitioner–patient relationship. This may stop wasteful considerations and a non-productive consultation. A psychosexual practitioner notes, 'It is a necessity to ensure safe and accountable practice; without this supervision the work becomes less efficient and consequently the number of times the patient is seen increases.'

Benner (1994) suggested that practice can be developed when practitioners study:

1. Situations where they felt successful and thought their intervention had made a difference.
2. Situations where they were not satisfied with their performance.

These two perspectives are particularly relevant in the advanced seminars where the members are more confident about their understanding of the work, thinking for themselves and not reliant on or expecting answers from the leader or the group. They are more relaxed about sharing feelings and can show excitement with successes; the pain continues to be experienced but, as one member said, 'perhaps one is not so fearful of it'.

Where the members of the group have not been satisfied with their performance they now have the strength to expose their weaknesses in a clinical presentation. Support and supervision from the seminar enables the members to show courage and have the confidence to initiate work with patients.

The practitioner is always listening and, from our experience, ready to modify responses to differing patients and events that are talked about. When the work is difficult, however, there is a greater likelihood that she will feel that she is not satisfied with her performance and will bring this consultation to the group.

The following story was told to a seminar group. The nurse felt a failure as she had not been able to offer the patient anything and could not understand the practitioner–patient relationship. The material presented was confused but also very painful for all concerned, the patient, the nurse and the group.

'An attractive 40-year-old woman with long, dyed hair came to see me by appointment for a psychosexual consultation. Very quickly she told me she had come because, as she said, "I have reduced libido and I have never had an orgasm with intercourse. I would like Viagra – if I was a man I would be impotent." My response was to be quite shocked and explain that Viagra was not available for women. "That's a pity," she said and went on to say, "I have always been cheated and I am never satisfied with sex." She had only come for help now because "I can't tell my present man, as he would leave me – like all the others. I have had so many lovers, if only they knew how impotent I am." She poured out a rambling story of physical and emotional abuse, and I felt unable to stop her also telling me of a poor relationship with her parents. We discussed this relationship and she told me "my parents disapproved of my boyfriends in adolescence and this has persisted with my male friends, so I rarely visit them, and now I regret this." Our time was up for the consultation but she left saying, "Perhaps I should try and see my parents again." We made another appointment. I was confused and overwhelmed by this story and I felt I had not been able to offer her anything.'

In the subsequent discussion, the group noted that the past history was heard but the presenting psychosexual problem and the focus of the practitioner's work was lost. One of the keys to understanding the presenting problem in a seminar is working with the here and now. It was commented that this did not happen, there was no discussion about the present boyfriend and their sex life together. The group also reflected on the overwhelming story and the painful picture of this woman's experiences with men, but there never appeared to be real connection of feelings. Was this a defensive detachment from the events by both? The presenting nurse realised she had failed in the obvious task of exploring the practitioner–patient feelings, and thought she herself had also become detached. The work had stopped. This nurse then said, 'How does this reflect my patient's experience of a sexual relationship with her present partner?' The group discussed how the nurse might be able to work in the next session with the patient, to look only at the present situation and the feelings that might be around between the woman and her partner.

The nurse described their next encounter at the following seminar (see Case study 18.3).

A member of the group reflected on this encounter and wondered if the word 'advanced' hampered the work sometimes and commented, 'perhaps we are afraid of being naïve'. In a seminar, working with the here and now is important (with all its naïvety), i.e. being able to stay with the psychosexual

Case study 18.3

'She arrived looking much happier and told me she had been to see her parents and felt some good changes had taken place in their relationship. "I was so pleased with myself and feel much stronger about seeing them again." Then she asked me, "But how is that going to change my sex life?" This made me think of our last seminar discussion and reflecting on this I was able to introduce the idea of her being detached from her feelings, and commented that perhaps this affected her ability to have an orgasm with her present boyfriend, because it seemed difficult for her to commit herself to any man. She answered quite crossly, "He isn't emotionally strong enough to hear what I have to say. I have always had to care and be responsible for the men in my life. I don't want him to leave me as I feel we do have a good relationship, apart from the sex."

At this stage we had begun to work together and our relationship changed to one of mutual respect. We began to discuss her feelings of anger and her vulnerability as a woman. She then told me, "But I can orgasm with the use of a vibrator which he gave me but I want to be normal like other women. I feel a failure and abnormal."

My recollection was of failure after the first consultation. I realised it was a mirror of her feelings and showed how powerfully she had led me away from the real problem and the avoidance of her painful feelings of anger and failure. I feel we have started to move a step nearer to finding a resolution to this woman's distress.'

problem and not to get caught up with the complexities. Practitioners are often trying to fit together the past and present, which causes the confusion for the patient and the nurse but it may also be crucial to the outcome of the consultation. This is clearly demonstrated in the above story. Where the practitioner recognises the need for counselling for other issues then an appropriate referral can be offered.

Responses to the advanced seminar

As with any Balint seminar training, the group will depend on the skills of the leader and the receptiveness of the members. The development of further skills can occur more quickly than in earlier training and the essential cohesiveness usually develops rapidly. It is not a new experience for the members to find a freedom of interaction. A supportive relationship develops where there is no mistrust or competition and there is an honesty in reporting the presentations. A practitioner wrote, 'It is a relief to share one's helplessness in the practitioner–patient relationship.'

Patients express the same relief sometimes when they say, 'I'm so pleased I have told you, I feel so much better.' The seminar is also a restorative process when interactive skills have disappeared and a period of disciplined reflection is required to understand why and how they were lost in that encounter.

Leadership skills

The leader is present to develop a greater depth of skills, drawing attention to the behaviour of the practitioner and the patient and the effect on their relationship. The members of an advanced seminar cannot afford to become complacent; at the same time they want to value their psychosexual work and share this experience with other practitioners. The leader may have to continue to draw attention to the defences that are used by patients and members of the group. A member of the group wrote in a self-assessment of her performance: 'one of my habitual dilemmas is to be able to distinguish between my "thoughts" and my "feelings".' The leader may have to draw attention to the failure to distinguish between thoughts and feelings in a practitioner–patient relationship. Balint group members would identify with this and it is a continuing dilemma for many practitioners.

The advanced group know that without a leader the focus of study and the feelings involved in practice would not have the necessary rigour. Space is available in a seminar to clarify the avoidance of work and provide a way to refocus and if necessary to reset the agenda with the patient. The following case study illustrates how a group member was able to refocus the work after presenting it to the seminar.

Case study 18.4a

'A GP referred a 34-year-old man to my psychosexual session and told me that this patient was having erections but was unable to have vaginal penetration and ejaculation with his partner. I have seen him for three sessions, I feel frustrated and fed up each time he returns, I don't really like him. But I realised after his last visit I had gone off on one of my old tacks, looking for a physical cause and not concentrating on our practitioner–patient relationship. I have brought it to the seminar because I am wondering how I can begin again?'

The leader and the group concentrated on the strong feelings of the practitioner being 'fed up'. The leader asked the group to identify where this feeling originated. A member suggested that it was from the patient, that he must be very fed up with not having satisfactory sex. The leader commented, 'you were both fed up, I would suggest' and reminded the group that practitioner–

patient relationship is concerned with staying with and understanding that relationship. Someone else suggested that perhaps the patient was fed up also with practitioner for not solving the problem. The practitioner realised she had neither stayed with the relationship nor understood the feelings that were around in this consultation and they were both fed up with the situation.

The presenting practitioner reflected on this discussion and described the fourth encounter to the seminar a month later.

Case study 18.4b

'Early in the consultation I was able to say, "You must feel very fed up with our lack of progress, perhaps it feels like your lovemaking? You are able to have great foreplay and then you are unable to get inside her." There followed a long silence – I had to wait, perhaps he was surprised by my recognition of one of his feelings?

At last he said, "You are right, I shouldn't put up with this one-sided relationship." We were then able to discuss how he felt she controlled their relationship. His irritation was explosive as he told me he was supposed to perform on demand. I knew then that we had refocussed the work and made a breakthrough when he could express his feelings about the situation. He left saying, "I am not going to perform on demand any more." At the next and last brief visit I hardly needed to ask, a big smile said it all.'

In this encounter the leader's role can be studied: she had to be aware of the feelings aroused in herself when listening to this story but also to consider how to throw light on the practitioner not being able to get close to the man initially, at the same time finding some illumination of that experience to help the practitioner feel supported and enlightened but not advised. In this story there was no condemnation of the feelings of the practitioner in not liking the patient. In the advanced seminar there is an acceptance of the patients we like to work with and those we do not like to work with. Having the experience and ability to make use of freedom of thoughts often enables practitioners to talk easily about emotions and sexual matters with patients. The practitioner can not only face the overt emotions but also has the skills to pick up concealed emotions and offer the confidence to the patient to talk.

A group member described the following patient who had come in for a blood test (Case study 18.5).

The group in the discussion commented on this member's sensitive approach, which gave Mrs P the confidence to talk about a hidden anxiety. There was no evidence from this encounter that she intended to raise her anxiety at that time. The group felt the member's psychosexual skills had been instrumental in allowing Mrs P to confide in her, with an opportunity to follow-up this inter-

---

Case study 18.5

'This lady, Mrs P, is 35 years old and I was taking a routine blood test. She suddenly started to tell me she had received 11 pints of blood following her sterilisation 18 months ago, which she described as having "gone wrong". I felt quite shocked and she appeared to be quite distressed; she obviously wanted to tell me something else, but hesitated. There was a short silence then she said, "Since that experience I cannot stand my husband being near me." I was quite surprised to be involved in her sexual life but I remember asking quietly, "I wonder what effect that has on your love making?" There was a long silence and eventually she said, "I have put him in an impossible situation, sometimes teasing him into having sex with me and then rejecting him." I realised I had uncovered a psychosexual problem which needed further discussion and time. I have offered her an appointment for next week.'

---

vention and perhaps make some resolution for the patient. It was also noted that, having the flexible approach and knowledge of an 'expert' (Benner 1984), she could pick up Mrs P's concealed emotions during her everyday practice.

These stories presented to the advanced seminar give a brief glimpse of the work encountered as psychosexual practitioners. They illustrate the variety of practice with its failures, complexities, sadnesses as well as excitements. The different relationships that are discussed, revealing feelings, become the essence of the study in a Balint seminar since they often illuminate the patient's anxieties and problems.

Joining an advanced seminar

Most of the members of the present advanced seminar joined at its inception but it is useful for educators to be reminded of the feelings of practitioners when they join a well established group. There are fears and fantasies about returning to a seminar and also the knowledge that in returning to the discipline of a Balint seminar there will be no escape from the rigour of practice. One member wrote:

It was hard for me to join an established group – all sorts of fantasies about myself appearing green and incapable paralysed my ability to present my own work for a while. Lots of learning from other cases was absorbed, where the sharing of pain, grief and successes became familiar again. Working as a psychosexual practitioner I had plenty of work to present and once I recognised that my fantasies were unreal then I could become fully involved in the training once more. Exciting and exhausting, but it is essential for my professional development.

Another member who had attended basic seminars in the past but more recently had gained skills on a counselling course and a different psychosexual training, joined the advanced seminar. These were her thoughts after 3 months in the advanced seminar:

I am with a group of people who have 'stuck' it out over a period of time, who have felt pain and joy, but keep going. There are no escapes of trying to find treatments or medication. I am secure in the knowledge that I have the strength to expose my weaknesses and difficulties without the fear that as an inexperienced member I may have to expose my own problems. The group is there to do the work and we do it, we are not there for our own personal therapy. I have experienced this in other trainings where personal problems have got in the way of the work. I feel very confident and relaxed in a setting where it has been spelt out that we are not there to discuss our own problems.

Joining the group as an observer/participant

There has been no formal research on the Balint seminars for practitioners. Recently, a nurse researcher joined the advanced group to conduct a pilot study of the training method. This had the full agreement of the seminar members, and the study is ongoing at the time of writing.

She writes of this experience:

As a researcher I am accustomed to being an outsider but in the seminar I feel warmly welcomed and drawn into the work with an immediacy that is very unusual. Having said that, I often find it difficult to pinpoint the feelings aroused by the group members' work, as channelled through case studies. The details of people's lives laid bare often prompt a flurry of emotion: compassion for the situations that people construct for themselves; unease, but also something more positive but difficult to name in recognising aspects of my own past in the presentations; fear of not speaking and not contributing to this joint project, detracting from the efforts of others; fear of saying the wrong thing, demonstrating my lack of understanding of the approach underpinning the seminar; admiration for the wisdom, perseverance and openness of the participants, their readiness to make themselves vulnerable; pleasure and affection in the frankness of their language, and the space they make for humour and spontaneity; sometimes puzzlement, in that I'm not sure where we are going. There are other times when I feel strangely drained of emotion, empty, as if untouched by the story. I think I am learning to see this as indicative of something in the nurse–patient relationship but I am intrigued by the extent of these emotional responses.

This outsider's view shows many of the anxieties that are experienced by seminar members in the early learning but also observes some of the skills of this advanced and experienced group of practitioners.

REFERENCES

Benner P 1984 From novice to expert: excellence and power in clinical nursing practice. Addison Wesley, Menlo Park, CA

Dreyfus H, Dreyfus S 1977 Uses and abuses of multi-attribute and multi-aspect model of decision-making. Department of Industrial Engineering and Operations Research, University of California, Berkeley (unpublished manuscript)

Conclusion

Diane Wells

This book was written for two groups of health care practitioners – those working with patients and those who coach the practitioners. Many readers may perform both these roles.

We have tried to show that certain features are common to both roles and a Balint approach to training emphasises the commonality. Health care workers endeavour to be alongside their patients in partnership. This feature of their work may be learnt experientially, not only through reflection on practice, but also in seminars where the leader tries to understand the practitioners by tuning in and being alongside their experience. When a practitioner values the leader's ability to get in tune with how she felt when with a certain patient, she can perceive how she also offers a similar skill to her patients. Perceiving the parallels between the teacher–learner relationship and the practitioner–patient relationship has been called the 'hall of mirrors' (Schon 1987). When the work is going well between practitioner and patient the mirror may be turned again to reflect on the patient–partner relationship.

In each dyad the model of partnership is observed, parallels perceived and the experience may be internalised. Yet the model taken away from the interaction by each patient, practitioner, or coach will be different. Each of them has a living example of the complex interplay of thought, feeling, experience and individual differences which occurs through the life span, as elucidated in the middle section of this book. When theories are demonstrated in this lively way it may be referred to as another form of reflection, because theoretical principles are reflected. This demonstrates a further value of returning to experience in thought, and with feeling, by telling the story. If practitioners' stories are valued by their teachers it is more likely that patients' stories will be heard and their meanings understood.

Just as the practitioner studies her relationship with her patients, so also the teacher or coach studies the group relationship she has with her students.

It is this study of relationships which is the hallmark of Balint seminars, distinguishing them from other forms of reflective practice. In a seminar where this study can follow the verbal accounts of clinical practitioners or seminar leaders, psychoanalytic principles of listening for the feelings help in the development of awareness and skills. Here again the principle is mirrored for the coach who studies her own group skills in a leaders' seminar.

The 'hall of mirrors' (Schon 1987), which is available in reflection, allows practitioner and coach to perceive their roles as part of a continuum rather than being separate and isolated from one another. This may be particularly valuable at a time when developments in health care education are perceived as having created an even wider gap between education and clinical practice.

Practitioners and teachers require support and training to continue developing interpersonal skills appropriate for each situation. Balint seminars provide training, the best form of support, and clinical supervision. If written accounts of interactions and seminar work are kept, as advised here, practitioners also have the basis for action research (Penman 1998).

Whether this book has been used to support your role as a clinical practitioner or as a teacher, we would like to continue working with you. There are plans for conferences and workshops to develop the themes of this book. In several places in the text the authors have mentioned regular Balint seminars for clinical practitioners, and leaders' groups. If you would like information on any of these current training opportunities, or future conferences and workshops, please fill in the form at the back of the book, and make copies for friends and colleagues. The first conference/workshop is planned for about 12 months after the publication of the book.

REFERENCES

Balint M 1957 The doctor, his patient and the illness. Pitman Medical, London

Balint E, Courtenay M, Elder A, Hull S, Julian P 1993 The doctor, the patient and the group. Routledge, London

Penman J 1998 Action research in the care of patients with sexual anxieties. Nursing Standard 13 (13–15): 47–50

Schon D 1987 Educating the reflective practitioner. Jossey Bass, San Francisco

Appendix: Short history of Balint training

Dr Michael Balint

Dr Balint was a Hungarian-born doctor, trained in psychoanalysis. He came to England in 1939 and worked in Manchester, particularly in child guidance. At the end of World War II in 1945 he moved to London, was appointed Director of a Child Guidance Clinic and practised as a psychoanalyst. A few years later he joined the staff of the Tavistock Clinic to train social workers.

Together with his future wife Enid, he evolved a scheme of training with regular group discussions related to people with marital problems. This led to the formation of the Institute for Marital Problems. (Hopkins 1987).

The development of Balint groups and training

Doctors were beginning to realize that there was a gap in their training, as patients were seeking help with their emotional problems and these were not described in the textbooks. General practitioners, in particular, were requesting some further training. Dr Balint placed an announcement in the medical press inviting doctors to attend the Tavistock Clinic for a 'Discussion group seminar on psychological problems in general practice.' The first training groups started in 1952. They were later called 'training-cum-research seminars' – a significant title – and are now simply called Balint groups. As a result of the work within these groups Dr Balint's book *The Doctor, his Patient and the Illness* was published in 1957. This research remains the seminal authority on this training.

The study

Dr Balint writes in his introduction to this book: 'thus we were faced with three different though interlinked tasks. The first was to study the psychological implications in general practice; the second to train general practitioners for this job; and the third to devise a method for this training.' He considered it was important to establish in the group 'a free, give and take atmosphere, in which everyone could bring up his problems in the hope of getting some light on them from the experience of the others. The material for our discussions was almost invariably provided by recent experiences with patients reported by the doctor in charge.'

The importance of the study of the emotional aspects of the doctor–patient relationship, he suggests, 'can only be obtained if the atmosphere of the discussion is free enough to enable the doctors to speak spontaneously.' Crucially, he states that 'the leader has to avoid as far as possible, the ever-tempting "teaching-being-taught atmosphere".'

The aim

The aim was to help doctors to 'really listen' and become more sensitive to what was going on consciously or unconsciously in the patient's mind. The training was established and recognised as being about the acquisition of a personal skill and that it would also require changes in the professional self. Here the doctors are enabled, within the group, to recognise the nature of their own approaches to patients. Those that might be useful can be developed but others that are not so useful, could be modified or, possibly, even abandoned.

There are Balint groups training worldwide, mainly in the medical field but with a wide focus of study from hospital-based care to community and family care (Journal of the Balint Society 1998, vol. 26).

The Balint Society

As a result of the work of these pioneer groups, the Balint Society was founded in 1969 to promote learning and continue research in the understanding of the doctor–patient relationship in general practice. Balint groups and workshops continue under their auspices for doctors and medical students (Balint Journal 1998).

Institute of Psychosexual Medicine

It was in 1960 that a group of doctors working for the Family Planning Association began to meet under the leadership of Dr Tom Main, then Director of the Cassel Hospital. He was a psychoanalyst with a special interest in group training. These doctors were finding that women requesting contraceptive advice were often seeking help with their sexual anxieties. Dr Prue Tunnadine writes in her Preface to *Contraception and Sexual Life:* 'Dr Main believes this therapeutic technique is taught and learned only by the living dynamics of clinical experience within the seminar system.' Main was referring to the members giving their account of the clinical event which was then to some extent relived and experienced by others in the group.

The Institute of Psychosexual Medicine was formed in London in 1974. The name was used to illustrate a therapeutic body–mind approach where the doctor makes use of listening skills and, when appropriate, physical examination. This approach continues to be used for the training of health care professionals. The Institute continues to train doctors from all disciplines of medicine.

Nurses' training

In the early 1970s family planning nurses were also becoming aware that their patients were requesting help for sexual anxieties. The nurses expressed a need for new clinical skills to deal with their own feelings of inadequacy and anxiety as well as those of their patients. As a result, the Department of Health and Social Services agreed to fund some experimental groups for 1 year initially. These were to help nurses understand psychosexual problems. Because of the success of these groups a second year of funding was sought and granted. The groups were led by a doctor in Birmingham and two nurses in London – Doreen Clifford, then Matron of the Cassel Hospital, and Juliet Wiltshire, Deputy Matron of the Maudsley Hospital. The group led by Doreen Clifford was a Balint-type seminar and the 13 nurses who formed the group worked mainly in family planning clinics in Central London (D Clifford, unpublished data).

Approved nurse training

The success of these groups led to the Joint Board of Clinical Studies (now the English National Board) approving a curriculum for a short course on the Principles of Psychosexual Counselling for Registered and Enrolled Nurses and Registered Midwives (ENB course 985). For 10 years between 1981 and 1990 the Balint seminar was incorporated into the training on the ENB 985 coordinated from the Olive Hayden Midwifery School, Lewisham Hospital. The course philosophy was: 'to enhance the nurses'/midwives' ability to recognise and respond to patients/clients presenting directly or indirectly with sexual anxieties. This includes a search for an understanding of normal human emotional development and the study of the nurse/patient relationship as a way of developing nurses' skills'.

Self-funding groups of nurses, midwives and health visitors continued to meet under the leadership of Doreen Clifford through the 1970s. From these groups, and from the ENB 985 course members at the Olive Hayden School, more leaders were trained, which enabled new groups to start. These still continue and are attended by nurses, midwives, physiotherapists and other health practitioners.

Other ENB courses have also integrated the seminar training into short courses, e.g. The Advanced Family Planning Course AO8 (Bell et al 1997).

Psychosocial nursing

Within the framework of psychosocial nursing, the Balint seminar has been used at the Cassel Hospital for the last 50 years. This hospital is a psycho-analytically based therapeutic community where there is a constant endeavour to turn the experiences into learning, using the everyday interaction of patients and staff as the focus of enquiry (Barnes 1998).

Many Cassel-trained nurses have been able to adapt the Balint approach for training in other fields of work. Wells (1998) uses this approach as part of the ENB course 'Nursing Elderly People' where 'biographical approaches to working with older people' are studied. The stories told by the patients are brought to the group by the practitioners. She writes, 'Balint-style seminars enable course members to discuss their relationships with their patients. These seminars provide nurses with time to express their feelings and to gain some theoretical understanding of these relationships.' About these relationships she comments, 'frequently, nurses want to discuss patients who are "difficult to nurse" but as the nurses tell their stories, they may be able to clarify thoughts and feelings, which, until that point, have been latent in their work.' The essence is in her conclusion: 'Biographical knowledge, however, is not enough; it is the relationship between the nurse and patient that is the crucial factor. It is here the nurse experiences tensions, responds to needs and gives support. When attention is paid to the emotional aspects of getting to know patients, nurses are best able to use a biographical approach in their care of patients'.

Others have used the seminars for the training of clergy, managers and educationalists. The common features of Balint seminars are:

◆ A leader
◆ A focus for study
◆ Discussion of the material and feelings in the relationship
◆ Reflection on practice
◆ Clinical supervision
◆ Action research.

The Association of Psychosexual Nursing

The Association was founded in 1998 by a group of nurses and practitioners who had been meeting informally for 10 years and had been trained in Balint seminars. These founding members felt committed to this training and wished to promote the Balint approach. The objects of the Association are 'for the relief of sickness and for the preservation and protection of public health by promoting and providing training for nurses and other health care professionals in psychosexual nursing, with particular reference to training methods as promoted by the Balint Society, with a view to maintaining and raising the standards of psychosexual nursing'. Full membership is open to those who are attending seminars or have been in seminars in the past. Subscribing membership is available to those who have an interest in the objectives of the Association.

REFERENCES

Balint M 1957 The doctor, his patient and the illness. Pitman Medical, London

Barnes E 1998 Preface. In: Barnes E, Griffiths P, Ord J, Wells D (eds) Face to face with distress: the professional use of self in psychosocial care. Butterworth-Heinemann, Oxford

Bell J, Rutter M, Selby J, Ward M 1997 Nurse-led family planning. Practice Nurse 14(4): 265–267

Hopkins P 1987 Michael Balint: the man and his work. Psychiatry in Practice November: 12–16

Tunnadine P 1979 Contraception and sexual life. A therapeutic approach Tavistock, London (out of print)

Wells D 1998 Biographical work with older people. In: Barnes E, Griffiths P, Ord J, Wells D (eds) Face to face with distress. Butterworth-Heinemann, Oxford

Index

CARING FOR SEXUALITY IN HEALTH AND ILLNESS
EDITOR DIANE WELLS with DOREEN CLIFFORD, MARJORIE RUTTER
and JANE SELBY

We plan to run conferences and workshops to continue the work discussed in this book. Please use this form to let us know how this book has been used and to inform us about your needs for ongoing training. If you would prefer to write a letter please feel free to do so.

RESPONSE FORM

NAME (capitals) _____

ADDRESS (capitals) _____

_____

OCCUPATION _____

PLACE OF WORK (capitals) _____

1) WHAT USE HAS THIS BOOK BEEN TO YOU, e.g. have you used it in relation to practice, teaching, or thinking about experiences?

2) WERE ANY CHAPTERS OF PARTICULAR VALUE? Please state how you have used them.

3) DO YOU THINK ANY PARTS OF THE BOOK COULD HAVE BEEN DIFFERENT? e.g. longer, shorter, simpler or more detailed?

4) DO YOU HAVE AN OPPORTUNITY TO ATTEND TRAINING SEMINARS TO SUPPORT YOUR PSYCHOSEXUAL PRACTICE OR TEACHING?

5) WOULD YOU LIKE INFORMATION ON SEMINAR TRAINING FOR PRACTITIONERS/LEADERS? (delete as appropriate)

6) WOULD YOU LIKE INFORMATION ON WORKSHOPS and CONFERENCES?

7) ANY OTHER COMMENTS?

PLEASE RETURN TO – ASSOCIATION FOR PSYCHOSEXUAL NURSES PO BOX 2762 LONDON WIA 5HQ, UK

DETAILS WILL BE SENT TO YOUR HOME ADDRESS UNLESS YOU INDICATE OTHERWISE